After Depression

After Depression

What an experimental medical treatment taught me about mental illness and recovery

GREGORY DOUGLAS HARMAN

ISBN-13: 978-1516854929
ISBN-10: 1516854926

About the Author

Gregory Douglas Harman is an independent journalist based in San Antonio, Texas. His writings have been published in *Guardian Sustainable Business*, *Houston Press*, *The Texas Observer*, *The Austin Chronicle*, *The Dallas Morning News*, and the *San Antonio Current*. He has been recognized for his investigative journalism and column writing by the Association of Alternative Newsweeklies, Houston Press Club, the Lone Star Chapter of the Sierra Club, and Public Citizen Texas, among others. He currently serves as a contributing editor at *Texas Climate News*. This is his first book.

CONTENTS

2. Beneath the 'Eggbeater'

Introduction

Depression advances along a million unique tracks shrouded behind a gallery of distortions. It sails to mind from an unfamiliar distance, picking apart confidence and undermining relationships as it weaves its way through one's mental and emotional body, calcifying there as a sort of malign superstructure. With time the victim comes to define their essential self by this colonizing force, this veritable subtraction of the self. And that is, perhaps, the greatest tragedy of this global epidemic.

Still poorly understood, the interlocking mechanisms encouraging the malady's growth worldwide are debated by researchers absorbed in the interplay of genetics, trauma, inflammation, and environmental exposure, among other factors. For those who suffer from it, harder than understanding the beast is getting out from beneath its grip, or—more realistically — living alongside it with any degree of self-compassion.

My own decades of depression and anxiety have been no different. In 2012, circumstances demanded that I prioritize recovery. I quit my job and joined an experimental device trial exploring the potentially depression-busting power of spinning magnets—a twist on increasingly common transcranial magnetic stimulation, or TMS.

Boston-based NeoSync's egg-shaped NEST device (shorthand for NeoSync-EEG Synchronized TMS), shows promise. Thanks to the design of the clinical trial, I have no way of knowing how many weeks of authentic treatment I received, but a paper published in in the journal Brain Stimulation earlier this year seems to demonstrate I was not the only one who benefited. "The study found sTMS therapy to be significantly more effective than sham when administered as intended, supporting the hypothesis that low-field magnetic stimulation improves depressive symptoms," wrote Andrew Leuchter, a psychiatry professor and director of the neuromodulation division in the Semel Institute at University of California, Los Angeles.

The study designed and funded by NeoSync and conducted at 17 sites around the country between 2011 and 2013 appears to be another validation of the growing interest in magnetic fields in the treatment of a growing range of brain disorders. The NEST, or "Eggbeater" as I came to call it, is far from a panacea. But for those who do respond, it is a potential lifesaver—should the U.S. Food and Drug Administration one day approve its use by the general public.

My hope is that this volume—the product of two years of exploration and experimentation built upon firsthand reporting and research and drawing on a collection of blog posts written through the clinical trial process —will serve as a resource and source of encouragement for fellow sufferers and those who love them. In addition to offering whatever insights my harder years have provided, I hope in some small way also to contribute to the destruction of the deeply damaging and misguided stigmatization of those who suffer from depression's drag and the broad array of mental intensities trailing along in its billowing cloak.

Portions of this book have been previously published by *The Austin Chronicle, Fort Worth Weekly, San Antonio Current,* and Depression-Time.com. It is dedicated to those who chose to love me these many years, difficult as that has been at times. And it is for those who have allowed me to love them in return.

I. Things as Things Are

Breathing in the Panic

If you desire healing, let yourself fall ill.

— *Rumi*

I'm grasping the top of the desk, whorls of white-creased joints trembling behind eight blood-drained fingertips, resisting the impulse to run. My entire biology screams for flight. Instead I freeze in place, oblivious to the blare of the music coming from the designer's desk just outside my door. I'm staring dutifully into an oversized Apple monitor like most of the editorial team scattered around the second floor of the weekly magazine office. I'm staring into stacked lines of text, carved out pecks and scratches running along furrows in a nonsensical rhythm. Somewhere in my core a wild shuddering threatens to surface.

I wheel in long, thin breaths as if from some distant well. The inhalation clamps down on the rising panic, compressing the rebellious tremors in my stomach, bearing down with the weight of desperate intention. Each exhalation softens my grip, allowing these layers of fear to peel away, a weightless moult drifting on the air. In again rushes fresh terror and another temptation for the will to crumple, to give in to what I assume would be irreparable madness. Another threading breath. Another tightening.

I've got to get the fuck out of here.

Perched at this endpoint of the productivity humming beyond my walls, I force myself to sit with the obligations and expectations of my position. After what feels like a respectable period of panic, I stand uneasily. Stumbling over the streaming cords at my feet, I push forward, walking just fast enough to avoid any interrupting signals from the staff. I have to instruct my legs not to run down the stairs, stairs to the exit sign and into the air. A small kinky-coated dog paces on the other side of the glass and watches me vanish beyond the parking lot and up the street as the Catholic school students meander distractedly to the assortment of trucks and SUVs waiting to carry them home. Terrified of being observed, I move down a set of limestone steps to the shaded path alongside the river. My breaths grow deeper and slower.

The air is thick with flower fragrance and the light and shadow dance above and across the winding waters. I hone my focus, hoping to rein in this quaking, these racing thoughts, with outward-directed attention. I'll cry, just a little, once, twice, as I plead with whatever power is beyond me. *What is wrong with me? Why am I not getting better?* Once or twice I'll retreat to old affirmations of a groundless faith, thanking a God for taking away my anxiety. Speaking things that are not as if they were. There are so many strategies.

My breath plants me in the present moment and I observe intensely, intentionally, the shape and rustle of trees, the near imperceptible movement of clouds, the sound of my feet sweeping over the cement path, the press of gravity, my embodied thickness. I repeat the Buddhist blessing, "May all sentient creatures everywhere be happy." I imagine my respiration as a wind filling not my lungs but my heart. It enters as through a curtain; it passes through in a prayer.

It's still a month before I will quit my job and slide a rope around my neck, seeking to silence the unbearable flashes of lightning-like panic, the terrible current buzzing like a jammed doorbell that rushes from mind to body, scrambling reality and reason. Right now, I am sitting by the water. I am crossing a bridge. I am on a dirt path. I am losing focus. I'm sweating. A barge moves by — I don't remember hearing it — and the water folds back, back upon itself, inverting the wall, the path, the bushes and trees of the opposing bank. I am losing focus. One fold into the next, water always changing hands in light, then hiding another emptiness.

I imagine falling beneath the dancing surface and

into its unreflecting fluidity, its meanderings imperceptible beyond the occasional snip of cottonwood leaf or disintegrating plastic. The dance is lifting sediment that shelters and soon buries the homes of river cooters and aluminum cans, engine parts and leaden fishing weights. Sometimes there are fish, their only evidence in the murk a sudden, audible redirection of the shimmering and streaming ripples traveling until they die, this way or another. One less insect sitting on the light.

A convincing teacher once said, "Suffering is the repeated unwillingness to accept things as they are." Internalizing that message, I made lists of everything I regretted, disliked, resented. Then I turned these surveys into chronicles of acceptance.

One read:

- *I accept completely who I am and take full responsibility for all my actions: good, bad, neutral.*

- *I accept that I am prone to panic attacks and suicidal bouts of depression.*

- *I embrace my heart, full to bursting with the desire for love, service, companionship.*

I return to a desk of tightly pressed and polished wood dust and glue, an object full of emptiness and poison. I answer a few emails. I watch a video. No one comes to my door. They only watch, warily, uncertain about the changes that have overtaken me these last months. This is how it's been since I gathered them together to tell them of my panic attacks, that I'd be cutting my hours and going into an outpatient mental-health program. A few will approach in the weeks to come to tell me of their secret struggles. There's a law of vulnerability at work here, a tender reminder of the life's indiscriminate hardness and our need for connection.

Perhaps such intimacies could have prevented this confounding obliteration of personal power. Perhaps if they had started years ago before my relationships began falling away in clumps with each job-related move. But there's a momentum behind these forces that can no longer be avoided or redirected. I'd talked about leaving my job at the news magazine for years, dispirited by an accelerating pace of staff dismissals, the ownership's apparent lack of interest in our news mission, and a constant low-level pressure to sell our readers on the hamburgers, nightclubs, and craft beers our advertisers promoted. But now? There was no more debate. I knew I'd have to leave, make way for someone still blessedly unsavaged by stress, one of those fortunates who had so far dodged this colliding symptomology. *Nothing is certain*, I think. *Everything is tenuous.*

But I've lost focus. I have to focus again.

Skirting Doomsday

It's about rebirth. Not death.

— Ricardo Agurcia, Maya scholar

So many doomsday predictions didn't come to pass in 2012. No supervolcanoes shook the earth or blacked out the sun. No sudden magnetic pole shifts wreaked havoc on GE, Telefon, Boeing. Sadly, no interstellar conquest came to subjugate our wayward species. A space rock fell, but it arrived two months late to a less-than-catastrophic result over Russian skies.

Yet when December 21, 2012, dawned on Texas — the widely publicized "last" day of the Mayan calendar — I was hemmed in on all sides, a defeated, humiliated wreck consigned to spending my days on the couch, moving unsteadily from room to room in an increasingly thick, pharmaceutical-induced haze. After

decades battling depression, an explosion of daily
panic attacks leading to a deepening despondency and
suicidality had brought me to the point of
psychological collapse.

Waking up each morning, I was forced to consider
that I could be disabled at 42. That this was as far as
my professional life would go.

It had taken months to get an appointment with a
psychiatrist after the panic attacks began the previous
spring. They were months I simply had to grit my
teeth through and force my steps to follow one after
the other. I'd been through it many times in my life,
convinced my attacks were malevolent spirits, psychic
attacks, premonitions about that black car down the
road. A man in a suit with a sniper's rifle with me in
his sights. Years upon years before I knew I had a
medical disorder, one familiar already to millions.

My new chemistry – the creation of daily doses of
Prozac, lithium, Wellbutrin, Klonopin, and sleeping
pills – felt like engaging the gears of a duller, more
drawn-out death. I became a strange creature to
myself, cautious, methodical, and distant. I holed up,
terrified of having to explain my sorry state to
acquaintances, watching old TV dramas in season-
spanning guzzlings. The only place I felt a sense of
belonging was at a downtown church basement and
homeless-services center I volunteered at. And that's
where things could have stalled for a very long time, as
they do for many diagnosed with a mental illness,
grudgingly coming to terms with newly restricted
abilities punctuated by periodic breakdowns,

medication tweaking, and dim hopes to one day be of use to someone again.

A suicide scare led me to the ER. Doctors were recommending electroconvulsive therapy, historically the treatment of last resort for those with major depressive disorder. But I already had my eye on something else, a experimental tweak on a magnet-based treatment I had written about two years earlier: a safer, noninvasive therapy known as rTMS, or repetitive transcranial magnetic therapy.

Introducing Magnets

The neuroplastic revolution has implications for ... our understanding of how love, sex, grief, relationships, learning, addictions, culture, technology, and psychotherapies change our brain.

– Norman Doidge, *The Brain That Changes Itself*

The first time I heard of magnetic therapy of any sort was years ago in Wyoming. I'd screwed up my neck. Couldn't turn my head without my muscles going into spasm ushering in incredible pain. A chiropractor gave me valerian root capsules to relax the muscles and suggested rounds of hot and cold therapy. A friend suggested a lodestone, a typically magnetic mineral known as magnetite.

"One polarity pulls tissues apart," he said, "the

other polarity makes them stitch back together." Alternating between the two would speed up healing, he said. He'd used it on his knee years ago. I never got a lodestone to experiment with, however, and it was a slow, uncomfortable healing.

Magnets have been used as medicine since ancient times and in a variety of cultures, including China and Ancient Greece. During the Middle Ages, magnets were prescribed for everything from baldness to arthritis. While modern science remains skeptical of many of the claims being made in alternative-health circles today, one clinical success appears to be the ability of magnets to help reduce arthritis pain. A frequently cited study at Houston's Baylor College of Medicine published in 1997 in the *Archives of Physical Medicine and Rehabilitation* found that 76 percent of post-polio patients suffering from arthritis reported relief after wearing low-intensity magnets over their sorest points. Significantly, only 19 percent of those who received the placebo reported improvement.

Magnets were used in the treatment of mental disorders in the West, to questionable effect, for hundreds of years before the rise of the pharmaceutical industry at the close of World War Two. Despite being sidelined by the rapid ascendence of biochemical interventions, magnetism still had contributions to make, including in the now-ubiquitous Magnetic Resonance Imaging diagnostic systems (which, researchers soon began to notice, exhibited anti-depressant qualities). That contribution is speeding up again. Critical to the magnet's re-ascendance is a new understanding of the brain's "plasticity," a recognition that both internal habits of thinking and outside forces can change the structure of the brain, even restore formerly clouded or diminished brain regions such as the dorsolateral prefrontal cortex, frequently implicated in the experience of depression.

I first witnessed the magnetic approach to depression treatment as a reporter in 2010. Walking into a nondescript San Antonio clinic I found a man with a football player's physique flirting with a Skittles-chewing lab tech. Then in his sixth week of TMS treatment, "Jay" told me how a quarter-century earlier he had been struck by a bolt of anxiety so powerful and inexplicable that he thought he was having a heart attack. The ER doctor, however, informed the deeply unsettled college student that he was simply too stressed out. He went home, but the panic attacks didn't stop.

"I ended up just going through and grinning and bearing it," he said. He had difficulty concentrating. His memory weakened. He obsessed over his deteriorating condition to the point that the undiagnosed anxiety disorder mutated into deep-seated depression. The only thing that kept him going was the belief that science would one day figure things out, that someone would invent a way out of his torment.

For him, that day arrived on December 16, 2008, when the U.S. Food and Drug Administration cleared Neuronetics' NeuroStar repetitive TMS device for medical use. Equipped with coils originally designed to treat incontinence, according to the health care newsletter *In Vivo*, the device was pitched as a safer, if less effective, alternative to electroconvulsive therapy. While the FDA panel deadlocked on that argument, it ultimately cleared the device on the basis of its lack of serious side effects and (as one member put it) "marginal" demonstrated effectiveness.

Overshadowing the FDA's clearance and perhaps loosening the standards for expected effectiveness was the Star-D study, the largest study of treatment-resistant depression ever undertaken. Published in November of 2006 in the *American Journal of Psychiatry*, the NIMH-funded "Sequenced Treatment Alternatives to Relieve Depression" study showed that even after multiple medications and behavioral therapy, modern psychiatric practice could only bring two-thirds of sufferers to full remission. It proved to be a major embarrassment to the psychiatric field.

This obviously wasn't the time to turn away even marginally effective alternatives. However, the health wing of the D.C.-based advocacy group Public Citizen protested the decision, suggesting that data showing the device was slightly better than treatment with a placebo had been manipulated to give the device the appearance of effectiveness. "It is concerning that FDA has cleared this device," the team wrote, "particularly if patients are diverted from effective therapies such as antidepressant medications."

Even with so little to recommend it, there were believers like Jay, who told me that after only his second treatment, TMS broke through his emotional dead zone and gave him a momentary glimpse of "normal" emotion for the first time in years. After more than a month of daily magnetic treatments, the man who estimated he had taken 15 different medications battling his entrenched illness, called TMS a "miracle," a "cure."

A Clinical Trial

What happens to the old when they cannot cross the last river?
Nothing. They stay behind to die. Only the dog is puzzled to see
a man abandoned.

— Miranda and Stephen Aldhouse-Green, *The Quest for*
the Shaman

Looking over my "Consent to Participate"
paperwork from the North Texas research hospital I
realize every page is marked with a "Do not Disclose"
stamp. I've been accepted for a clinical device trial
exploring the possible beneficial impact of an
electromagnetic device developed by Boston-based
NeoSync utilizing what the researchers were calling
"synchronized" transcranial magnetic stimulation, or
sTMS. Among the definition of terms in the trial
paperwork I see "Electro Convulsive Therapy" and

I'm grateful once again that this procedure will not be that. ECT had been recommended during my time in outpatient therapy when it seemed that whatever drug they threw at me failed to diminish my desire to disappear. "Memory loss isn't a huge issue," one psychiatrist would tell me later, "except maybe for writers or people who rely heavily on their... *What is it you do?*"

Despite ECT's advertised recovery rate of 80 percent, my memory was weak enough as it was. And the idea of resting beneath subtle waves of low-level magnetism was significantly more attractive than submitting myself to a series of electrically induced seizures while under general anesthesia. There was really only one other option besides the trial: taking (most of) the pills I was on now and going back to work at a less demanding job. Whatever I could manage. Perhaps a line cook oblivious to hot grease and grill burns, or (better) re-shelving books at a local library in a quiet contemplation. Inevitably, an ego rises behind such thoughts, resenting the loss of whatever public regard journalism allows writers and editors. Strange, I think, that I would feel such affinity with a career ranked as the worst job in the nation due to factors like stress, income, and hiring outlook. Somewhere between 2014 and 2015, it replaced lumberjacks at the bottom of the stack. *Ah, well.*

What to do when your dreams run into a new impermeable reality? Do you adapt or splatter yourself against this new boundary wall? Even if this so-called synchronized TMS moved me somewhere higher and more functional, I couldn't help but wonder who I'd be without my depression enfolding me. What comes after depression? Despite its interest in isolating and extinguishing me, depression's bottomless recess has been a reliable colleague and confidant insulating me from the world in its indifferent, unreachable absence.

Tapering off my meds with a month before the six-week trial opens, I pull the blankets tighter around myself, position my feet atop the electric floor heater. It does little to cut the chill in this 1930s plaster-walled bungalow when it approaches freezing outside. Mood disorder or no, any enthusiasm about what's to come is kept in check by this frigidness and complementary fever. Thank the Good Graces there is a darling companion to deliver fruit, warm lemonade with cayenne, and long, tender embraces. That alone makes this wait tolerable. She's unambitious in our commitments to one another—perhaps because of the nature of the relatable madness that stalks us both—asking only that I allow her to love me.

Underwater

It's only when hope disappears ... that enduring stress becomes true suffering.

— Sukie Miller, *After Death*

Imagine waking up with a start at the bottom of the ocean, say facing 11 kilometers of water from the floor of the Marianas Trench. There's a crushing weight of water above you and no chance of breath. Strangely, you don't die. Yet this screaming realization of imminent doom drags on without softening, a shock that should dissipate but doesn't. There is nothing but the terror exploding inside you.

My first panic attack hit at fourteen. Racing through the house, I could only grunt out garbled syllables and gesture frantically when I found my mother at the back door. Confused and fearful, she drew me to the rocking chair in the front of the house and sang to me until the attack passed. For that moment I was six years old again, wilting into a slow stabilization. It would be more than decade before I began to understand what had happened. This strange haunting would return with an increasing frequency in the years to come, especially the more I drank to keep the anxiety in check. Alcohol, one of the first prescriptions for such nervous disorders, failed miserably.

This wasn't where my mental-health issues began, but it was close. I'd love to be able to draw a stark straight line from this confounding turbulence to a solitary causative agent. For years, early sexual trauma was my favorite suspect. While friends in the neighborhood were sexually abused by a man just two houses down the sloping hill leading to the Little White Store (later becoming the Little Green Store following a new paint job) where we all stocked up on candy and soda, I've only ever had what I can call "body memories" suggesting I had been involved. Years later, there was a period of missing time when a man who picked me up hitch hiking made a wrong turn and then drove around in circles. There may have been a tunnel. I can't recall. In any event, I didn't make much progress in my search for stability until I stopped asking the question, stopped the obsessing and the attempted guided regressions led by the therapists I saw, and turned my energies to actively changing my ways of thinking via an evolving cognitive therapy developed in response to gathering recognition of the plastic nature of the brain.

The mind can be retrained, I came to understand, but it doesn't reprogram overnight. You've got to be disciplined, down for the long haul, and make use of all the tools at your disposal. Meditation? You bet. Exercise? Uh huh. Good diet? Check. Talk therapy. Yep. Meds? When recommended. A social life? Some connection to others. And, yeah, there's an increasing array of technological fixes, including implants, induced seizures, magnets. I'm warming up to it.

Shower Duty

All philosophies, however divergent they may sometimes be in the answers they bring, promise us an escape from primitive fears.

— Luc Ferry, *A Brief History of Thought*

"Why you so shaky? I make you nervous?"

The woman wasn't particularly menacing but she had an edge of confrontation to her voice. In several months of weekly volunteering in the basement of this downtown church I had never seen her before. An unknown quantity, she stepped closer to me as I produced the sign-in sheet for the women's showers.

"You want to talk to me or you want to take a shower?" I was trying to close the conversation, instead it led to more.

It was only 9:30 in the morning and I was already done with the day. I'd already gotten almost 40 men through the showers in time for breakfast in time to mop out the five stalls again with a strong bleach solution to get them ready for the women. I held jackets and traveling packs, riffled through the underwear box for better sizes, disappointed universally with our selection of ankle-high socks, and directed countless folks to the clothes "closet" down the hall. I felt like crap, to boot. Effects of the slow wean-off were definitely starting to show.

Was I shaking? I didn't know. Was this aggression or a simple question? I wondered as her friend accosted a church employee down the line, accusing them of "making a living off the church."

"Well," I started as her friend ambled over, "I have a major depressive and anxiety disorders and I'm going off my meds, so maybe that's it."

"Ha! He definitely sound like he's one of your people!" her friend cackles.

"I've got PTSD and major depression and anxiety," the first says, holding my fingers lightly. "So I feel ya. I feel ya."

Then turning from the hallway darkness, she continued: "But I don't take any of them meds they give you, cuz they have side effects. I just use chiva. That works fine for me."

They were headed to the dope house for a heroin fix after the showers.

Seizing Brain

Domestic disturbance. Man with golf club pounds on washing machine in garage. Woman in lawn chair applauds his every blow, whistles, barks like a dog. ... Officers linger in Patrol Unit, assess scene, swiftly reach unspoken agreement, gun engine, hightail it out of there.

— Daniel Orozco, *Orientation*

Night before last I took my last dose of Prozac. One result is a distinct sense of waking up. During a drive to the grocery store yesterday, for instance, I caught myself thinking how "normal" I felt. Would I be booted from the trial if these bright patches continued? It was a concern lasting for an hour, maybe two, before the next manic moment, which is to say: not very long. I still break down into tears dozens of times a day. Not tears moving me along any stages of grief, but tears of hopelessness and abandonment that have no bottom, no end until exhaustion sets in. Weaning off the pills, I also sense a fraying of the nerves. I'm short-tempered and slowed by a thought-congesting fog. Ugliness rises inside of me and festers in rumination and condemnation.

In the kitchen, my partner is pressing me, demanding an explanation for another of my sudden shifts in mood. She senses an intentional distancing, a rejection. I'm searching for words that will soothe her in my disordered state and find only a wild preverbal confusion. This failure of faculties, a strange and stunning inability to frame a simple idea, leads me to explode in frustrated rage. With homicidal force and an open-throated roar, I'm banging a pot full of rice and water against the range top. Then suddenly, inexplicably, the rage is replaced with a clarity, tranquility even. Stunned by the event, I stand dumbly, pot dangling from a limp hand, wondering at my violence. Of course, my partner, my anchor, has fled. I'm left alone to wipe the grains off the floor.

In these swings of beastly furies to periods of remarkable self-possession and optimism, the weeks stretch out. If I had bothered to thumb back a year back in my journal, or two years, or three, I'd see this roller coaster of stabilization and withdrawal was typical. One entry finds me talking about clouds lifting and a "departure from depression," and the next records an onset of sleeplessness and sorrow and "crazy thinking." When this particular round of anxiety began gathering a year ago, I dreamed of a home ransacked, lamps, books, chairs strewn around and piled in disjointed heaps. Digging through the chaos I discover dozens of laboratory vials packed with gelatinous eggs. Suddenly they begin to wriggle and hatch and streams of baby turtles, symbols of earth power I'll later realize, are winding toward me. A newborn parrot, illumination from the sky, zips in a colorful arch and lands on my finger. It dawns on me, I'm going to have to raise all these creatures myself.

After the rice explosion, my lover calls to check on me. She's back the next day, I have no idea why. But her faithful encouragement finds an echo during one of my sadly infrequent visits with my daughter. She knows a bit about what I'm going through and about the clinical trial before me. "Dad, I'm so proud of you for everything you're doing!" She repeats herself as I drive her back to her boarding school after our night out for dinner. I tell her again that she is the one who has given me the courage to persist again and again, to keep trying. In those hundreds of moments when living seemed the harder option, it's been my love for her that has sustained me.

Psychiatry's Failure

In the face of danger, we need to cleave together, becoming a new, many-headed creature larger than our individual selves.

— Barbara Ehrenreich, *Blood Rites*

As I've sought to understand my condition I've come to read a good share of books on psychology and evolutionary biology. The former have helped bring me up to speed with current research, the latter have driven home fear's deep roots. Just as we remain in some hidden pockets of the planet today, our ancestors hundreds of thousands of years ago were a prey species. Before we stepped out of the trees and onto the African savannah, we were huddled together in the high foliage chattering about movements of snakes and cats as the night fell.

That fear-response remained critical after entering

the plains and encountering the massive saber-toothed cats who proved unimpressed by our huddling and noisemaking. This long and traumatic family history loaded with its primitive fears is reflected in the deep position of the hypothalamus, the portion of the brain linking the endocrine and nervous system responsible for alerting the body to danger. These alerts manifest more often today in interpersonal conflict than any tangling with bloody-toothed predators. Full-blown anxiety attacks can be brought on by sustained periods of low-grade stress or even purely philosophical existential fears unknown by our ancestors. Panic attacks are what happens when that fight/flight switch gets stuck in place. Gaining power over it, getting "unstuck," takes a lot of training in recognizing the onset of anxiety before it escalates. And, yes, there are pills too for more immediate relief.

Characterizing one of depression's most obvious expressions, psychologist Rollo May famously called the illness an "inability to construct a future." The reason for that failure, however, is a cloudy one. We know that it's linked to heredity and the genes. But it also may involve toxins we increasingly pick up in our industrial environment. It's long been linked to trauma and abuse and more recently to the immune system and inflammation. Depression is, in other words, a many-headed hydra.

Yet psychiatrists still often seek to steer recovery by moving their patients from one pill to another. They teach us essentially nothing about the full range of contributors to our suffering or the many paths to recovery, many of which have been mapped out for centuries. Psychologists and therapists frequently send their clients scurrying after hidden histories and long-forgotten (and sometimes imaginary) shames at the expense of simple cognitive techniques that could help them manage their day-to-day distortions.

At an annual conference of the National Alliance on Mental Illness (NAMI), University of Tennessee assistant professor of psychiatry Dr. W. Clay Jackson issued a stirring critique of rampant "biological reductionism" dominating his field and urged a shift to a more comprehensive response to depression treatment. "I think we've made two grand mistakes in approaching mental health in this country, maybe three," he said. "One of those grand mistakes is we have stigmatized persons who have mental illness and we have separated it from biological illness." In recent years the medical establishment has overcompensated for that body-mind separation by making it all about the pill.

In a sweeping overview of depression and its treatments, Jackson made stops at Hippocrates, whose "black bile" of melancholy "comprises all fears and despondences if they last a long time," and Robert Burton's *Anatomy of Melancholy*, which prescribed a healthy diet, meaningful work, proper sleep, music, and time with friends, all of which (well, the type and volume of music may matter) are finding clinical support today. "Burton hadn't learned about St. John's Wort," Jackson said, "which would have been a wonderful addition to his book, but he didn't get out much," Jackson said.

That lack of exploration meant Burton also hadn't discovered Nidra yoga, which leads practitioners into a deep state of relaxation just this side of sleep, increasing dopamine generation as much as 65 percent, according to a 2002 study.

Sigmund Freud delivered the notion of childhood to Western minds, allowing for an understanding of childhood trauma—which we now know is a critical element loading the gun for depression. While German psychiatrist Emil Kraepelin is a hero of psychiatry for making way for groundbreaking contributions in how the human body relates to mental illness, his "tragic flaw," according to Jackson, was in leaving in the dust 5,500 years of accumulated depression-related wisdom.

"It's led to an explosion of pharmacotherapeutic options, but it's led to a relative paucity of non-pharmacologic options for patients to follow – or at least non-traditional, non-allopathic options," Jackson said.

There is no single depression gene. "There are probably 1,700 depression genes and they all interact," he said. And even then it is the environment and "early life adversity" that is believed to turn them on or off. That early destabilization creates an atmosphere of inflammation that causes the immune system to go rogue, leading often to a raft of health issues like hyperglycemia and weight gain. It puts people in a fragile emotional state so that events of seemingly mild significance send them into a tailspin.

And, he added, that depression may over time damage the brain's glial cells, responsible for clearing out glutamate—neurotoxic in excess—from the brain.

Finally, depression causes the hippocampus to shrink, making the hypothalamic-pituitary-adrenal axis less effective and less able to put the brakes on the stress response, leaving damaging cortisol to flood the body. The illness, he said, is probably neuro-degenerative in its final stages.

"There's a reason depressant patients feel more pain," Jackson said. "There's a reason they have more illness or sickness behavior. There's a reason they have fatigue. It's like they have the mother of influenza all the time. Their inflammatory processes are rampant."

Racing Depression

Black care rarely sits behind a rider whose pace is fast enough.
— Theodore Roosevelt, *Ranch Life*

In addition to being a conservationist hero and a racist Indian hater, President Theodore Roosevelt was a manic depressive. He was an avid hunter who knew what it meant to be stalked in turn by a force he referred to as "black care." To stay free he kept himself as busy as possible. It's a strategy I've heard others employing to some benefit. So as I move toward phase two of my recovery project by resettling at my parents' house, I strive to create a new groove full of volunteer work, exercise, and study, in addition to my experimental sTMS brain washing. I consider what it may mean to ride fast. There are boxes of books and journals piled before me. In spite of my preparedness,

I realize it's possible this search doesn't even develop into a story worth telling. At least, I think, I'll be keeping busy. At least I'll be making one last attempt to outrun my black care.

Rape Dream

We are such stuff as dreams are made on, and our little life is rounded with a sleep. Sir, I am vexed.

— *The Tempest*, Act Four, Scene One

Dream on returning to my parents' home:
A mother, a daughter, and a moderator sit together.

Moderator: So many people are making up these abuse stories because people want something for nothing.

Daughter: (Nods agreement)

Mother: (Turning to daughter) How can you agree with that considering what happened?

Daughter: I don't like to talk about the incident.

Mother: There was no incident. You were raped!

I dream I wake up and am relating the dream to

my loving partner, now sleeping beside me. I explain I
was represented by the mother, she by the daughter.
I'm barely getting the words out before my throat is
constricting and I'm choking on my tears. I remember
that in dreams every character represents another
aspect of the dreamer.

I wake.

Me: Did I tell you my dream?

Vulnerabilities

That is all I want in life: for this pain to seem purposeful.
— Elizabeth Wurtzel, *Prozac Nation*

Last night I dreamed of reptiles again. I had left them abandoned in paper cups and lousy cages, apparently, and spent most of the dream finding better, cleaner, newer containers, as well as food for them. Conditions seemed to be improving. On a final survey, I see one of the tanks is filled with gecko-sized baby elephants walking around and realize these are too complicated for me. For these I'll have to consult an expert like a wildlife rehabilitation specialist. Some situations require expert assistance.

Meanwhile, I'm tensing up every time I hear steps in the hallway. Terrified of being observed in my current state. Is my mom walking back to see me? Is my dad going to hug me again? Will they ask how I am while silently scanning me for signs of my illness or regretting they gave birth to such a troubled son? (Am I dressed? Am I shaved? Do I meet their gaze normally? Speak in complete, articulate sentences?) I am vulnerable before them in ways I hadn't anticipated. More than I'd like.

The fear is likely amplified by my disengagement of anxiety-reducing Klonopin, the last drug to drop from the roster. I've checked with the trial doctors. I can keep taking my fish oil and multivitamins, but no St. John's Wort, no brain-calming hormones. I can see what's coming. I see panic returning. Although they demonstrate an infinite patience, the gentlest acceptance, the psychic disassembling that full-blown panic represents is not an experience I long to share with my parents. I'm terrified of validating their most troubling anxieties, of causing them more grief. How I long to foster in them a belief that I'll soon be fine and self-sufficient. That I'm happy and at peace with the world. All the things that aren't yet true.

Dark Corners

There is always one moment in childhood when the door opens and lets the future in.

– Deepak Chopra

In my life I have made snow angels. And drank hot cocoa. And slid down hills. And bounced on the city's rubber reservoir cap in speedlace combat boots. I've driven too fast drunk behind night-vision goggles. I've smoked harsh chemicals through aluminum foil. I've also been sung to sleep, held hands at the zoo, kicked a perfect spiral, soaked in sights and smells and sounds many never have the opportunity to experience. And I've done kindness to others. In other words, I've had plenty of chances. One year there was so much snow we made tunnels through it without breaking the surface. I think that was the winter the sun-reflecting snows burned my retinas and I didn't notice.

I remember kissing behind the green kindergarten reading chair, chasing a dog as large and soft and white as a summer cloud. I remember covering my desk with a microscope set and notecards, thinking I'd be a brain surgeon one day. Or, surrounded by a pile of plush stuffed animals, a veterinarian. These are the flashes of childhood that come to mind when I cast back for a sense of happier times. A time before this. They are, however, mere snapshots of memory linked together in blank mystery. They are timestamps drifting in a forgetful sea. I remember getting older, though. Angrier and sicker. Thanks to my depression-damaged brain, many of the new memories fall out too. Only two brittle hands hold me now, guiding me, perhaps, down into the world of the hungry ghosts.

Choking

Caught at a distance from myself/ and there was no one there to know

— "Spring," Rites of Spring

What was the rope about? The one wrapped around my neck, twisting into my skin and forcing shut my airway and carotid artery? As I knelt a couple paces away from shelves of religious and spiritual books — lots about Buddhism and meditation, a large turquoise Bible, and yoga instructions (nothing, apparently, useful for this moment) — I looped the slick red-and-white camping cord around my neck a second time.

In those cold months before joining the trial, before de-medicating, I leaned my body closer to the floor and the quivering line running over the top of the bathroom door's hinge, secured on the other side by a dishwashing wand, grew still. My face swelled. Eyes and cheeks pulsed with such deep throbs I thought my skin would crack. A buzzing everywhere as my body lightened — all of my weight seemingly falling into my stretched, blood-bloated face. Then I sat up. I got some air. And did it again.

I'd been pacing room to room for over an hour, shaking in tantrum and falling into contorted shapes on the floor, howls rattling from my center as I searched the house for a solid anchor point, crouched in the attic. For rope. Something to separate my brain from my body, something to sever the connection between this erupting brain from the body it fills with a feral confusion, winding, consuming. Then I'm thinking of my daughter. It always comes back to my daughter. Exhausted, I release the rope as silence descends. A dull mind pooling on the floor. Quiet, quiet. Thoughtless silence. Just breathing.

Was this a suicide attempt or merely rope-play? How I interpreted it depended on my immediate psychiatric need. An affirmative response got me the outpatient care I needed early in my dysfunction. A denial allowed me into the sTMS trial. Those overseeing the study on NeoSync's behalf are concerned with the event. During a two-hour screening they seek to determine if I am certifiably depressed, specifically suffering from major depressive disorder (that's a requirement). They want to be certain I'm not schizophrenic, OCD, or actively suicidal.

I don't know it at the time, but they're also screening out those with eating disorders, ADHD, bipolar, drug addictions, obsessive compulsive disorder, and those with psychotic tendencies, multiple sclerosis, or dementia, among other conditions.

If the ropes were a severe state of despair — that is, "intensely despondent, 'experimenting,' or having an episode," according to the screening language — then it's OK. As one of my overseers puts it: If I had been aiming a gun at my head but then chose to shoot the ceiling at the last minute, that's not a suicide attempt. If I shot myself and still survived, well, that's a botched job.

II. Beneath the 'Eggbeater'

Lonely Train

There is a lonely train/ Called the 3:10 to Yuma/ The pounding of the wheels/ Is like a mournful sigh

— "3:10 To Yuma," Frankie Laine

I'm on the train headed to the hospital an hour away from The Decision. But even capitalizing the outcome of my noon meeting with the trial's chief investigator is to give the coming verdict too much weight. While I allow it's possible the experimental treatment could catapult me into new emotional territory, tease my neurons into making happy chemical signals, it likely won't. The chance of an outright healing, a "miracle" cure is such a long shot that it'd be ridiculous to pile all my chips on it.

The most likely outcome of the treatment, I've been told, is an improved receptivity to pharmaceuticals, a re-sensitization allowing one to reduce the number of pills they take, allowing a reduction of dosage. Off all my pills, life moves faster, comes with sharper angles. I have to rest frequently to maintain an ability to roll with this expanded sensory load. Trial or no trial, I tell myself as we hurtle past homeless camps sandwiched in the slices of greenery between the tracks and the highway, this rediscovered ability to regulate my moods has been worth the detour. A chance to step away from the medicines has shown I'm not irrevocably broken. It's been worth the season of unemployment and boredom. Facing down the vicissitudes of medication withdrawal. Leaving my house and my cats. Now I'm anxious to start rebuilding. To find a new job, a new career direction, new commitments to place and purpose. This, the person I am and the abilities I possess, is enough. It'll do.

Judging from the Bible quote staring at me from her desk, The Decider is a Christ-loving woman. She proved not completely adverse to — though, perhaps, not terribly adept at — potty language. Endearing herself to me forever, she offered a novice's invention: "shitola crappy." Did the rope experience make me feel "in control," she asked. Was it something I had thought about beforehand?

Synchronized TMS

The real vision ... is very real. It hits you sharp and clear like
an electric shock.

— *John Fire Lame Deer, Lakota holy man*

Synchronized transcranial magnetic stimulation,
evokes a hundred women in electrified flowering
bathing caps raising perfectly sculpted legs over the
water line and around their partners' shoulders as a
shimmering Fred and Ginger tap across a
revolutionary new plastic and glistening balls of
polyethylene-based polymers spin in the sky to the
tune of "My Sharona." That's what I'm expecting
from treatment. Just for the record.

sTMS involves three spinning magnets timed to stir
magnetic waves across the entire cerebral cortex at a
frequency unique to one's own alpha brainwaves—

typically between 8 and 12 cycles per second—in the hopes of restoring its normal electrical patterns. "Research has shown that the neuronal activity in the brains of people with depression shows abnormal brain rhythms in areas associated with depressive symptoms," said Mahendra Bhati, assistant professor of clinical psychiatry at Penn State University, in a press release promoting that university's trial, one of 15 others like mine taking place around the country. "sTMS therapy is based on the theory that the brain rhythms can be 'tuned' to a normal resting rhythm using low energy magnetic fields synchronized to an individual's brain activity. It is believed that this will restore normal brain rhythms leading to a reduction of depression symptoms and improved mood."

An article published in *Frontiers of Neuroscience* the year of the trial with the help of one NeoSync employee suggests that restoring those oscillatory rhythms along the brain's surface could actually positively impact deeper brain regions—including the thalamus and hypothalamus—by exerting "top-down control over broadly distributed brain regions."

Alone, these surface oscillations have been linked to everything from memory and mood to neurotransmitter levels and blood flow, all critically important in the experience of major depressive disorder. However, depression is also increasingly understood as a failure of the various brain regions to communicate effectively with one another. "Many of the mood and neurovegetative symptoms, as well as deficits in cognition and memory, have been hypothesized to arise from dysfunction in networks linking cortical and subcortical gray structures," the authors state.

In other words, the sTMS approach involves correcting "aberrant" alpha activity to "reset" deeper energetic oscillations, resulting in the "reemergence of normal, intrinsic oscillatory activity" and "possibly enhancing neuroplasticity, normalization of cerebral blood flow, and amelioration of depressive symptoms." The hope is this treatment will get the brain's energy circulating — rhythmically "oscillating" — properly again.

At the hospital, three electrodes are stuck to my head atop a shot of conductive jelly. Two go up front, one in the back. Yes, I'm told, the alpha waves are still wiggling. Apparently not everyone's are detectable. Another win for me. There's also an extended psychological battery of computer-generated questions about shapes and numbers and geometric sequences. And, finally, I'm informed my pharmacological history checks out. Lots of meds, lots of relapses or strike-outs. In other words, I qualify. First treatment? That would be Monday.

Drinking in Hell

Gather around me, Oh! ye death-defiant, and the earth itself shall be thine, to have and to hold!

— Anton Lavey, *The Satanic Bible*

Theme of this nightclub was Hell. Yeah, the place. But we still couldn't stay. Not past 2 a.m. In other words, there were still rules here. Black-clad and bloody, I watched patrons at the bar start ordering their murky thoughts and turning slowly toward the door.

Unlike the belligerent barking of "Bar's closed! Get out!" employed by some watering holes (some of which even pipe in the repulsive strains of the cowboy ballad "Happy Trails" to rouse the last of the drunks from their recesses inside black pleather booths back by the mistreated bathrooms) this proprietor's succinct message was brief and gracious.

"Thank you for coming. We'd love to keep partying with you. But you're not dead yet."

Then I woke up.

It was the closing scene of a night's worth of strange projections. There was an arching walkway like the St. Louis Arch not five feet wide dropping into a college football stadium to travel and critique. There were rude patrons at the food court to quibble with. A trip into the drinking quarter. Loose dogs. And then Hell.

It was a lot to wrestle with on waking so I focused on the conclusion. It proved easy to retain. "You're not dead yet."

In 30 minutes I headed over to the hospital for my first sTMS therapy session. The hope is it will revive my sluggish-to-dormant neurons at the front of my gray matter. That I'll see a return of feelings of pleasure and satisfaction. Worst case scenario is a headache … and possibly, if extraordinarily unlikely, seizure. If I don't notice anything new or unusual going on after a few weeks of Monday-to-Friday sessions that may mean I got the placebo—or that sTMS is a crock.

Under the Device

Together we're a chu-chi woo-chi, ooo-chi coo-chi pair/
Whatever you may ask becomes my happy task

— "Chu Chi Face," *Chitty Chitty Bang Bang*

I'm on my back in a dimly lit room on the seventh floor of the hospital. A device roughly two feet tall resembling an oversized egg is wheeled up behind me, its single blue clawlike appendage nestled possessively over the top of my head. "How's that?" the doctor asks.

A thumb drive containing my information is inserted, and a man's tinny voice buzzes from within the plastic shell announcing that a session is available. "Lie still with your eyes closed. Treatment begins in five, four, three, two, one. Treatment begins now."

Rattalattarattalattasqueeeeak! Rattalattarattalattasqueeeeak!

Rattalattarattalattasqueeeeak!
Low lights, an old massage table, and three spinning magnets. In a world seemingly awash in chemical solutions and all the hardship that has come to entail, here is the tentative rise of bioenergetic medicine. In the six-week, double-blind study, neither I nor the doctor administering treatment know if the ergonomic appliance vibrating on my head is generating a potentially therapeutic magnetic field or merely rattling in place.

"OK. I'll be back to check on you," says the lab-coated doctor with long, springy curls calf-length leather boots, as she drifts past a sign warning of strong magnetic fields.

I'm to keep my eyes closed but not fall asleep. The hope is that the energetic boost delivered by that magnetic field will stimulate patches of my brain that have grown quiet, if not dormant, stilled by decades of drug-resistant depression. I try to imagine what these awakened neurons – transmitters that in healthy brains communicate things like happiness and pleasure – would mean, before cursing myself quietly, as depressives will do, for thinking things could be different.

Nocturnal Struggle

How fortunate the son who finds in this immense world of objects one whom he can love, and, in loving, can regain his capacity to believe.

— Donald Capps, *Men, Religion, And Melancholia*

Her face in mine: calm, reasoning, fixed.
Mine in hers: angry, loud, wet lips spitting ugly demands.
Explain yourself!
I don't recall the exact words, the issues, or even the disagreement. But I recognize in the night's dream a younger me of barely bridled anger. As I wake up next to my partner (blessed be me for her tenderizing visits) I see something more important than a reminder of my defining '80s-era rage. I see that buried forces work to overwhelm me with anxiety even while I sleep. This

imbalance operates around the clock.

Lying under the white sheet and comforter, the shock of my partner's newly dyed fire-engine-red hair on the pillow beside me, I silently work like a taffy winder pulling apart the dream-born anger from this waking reality.

Did we really fight? No. One gauzy layer is drawn back.

Have I been betrayed somehow? No. Another layer, another degree of anger, lifts.

Is there someone else? Some injurious lie?

No and no.

The dream is reminiscent, I realize, of the fights I've had with friends and lovers past. But even after the reasoning mind has dispensed with the question of cause, the heat remains, the anger simmers on as my partner sleeps, innocent, of course, unaware of this fight that never occurred. I have to sit with the feeling and observe. And wait.

This afterburn doesn't require a reason for being. It just is. Like a living organism, it seeks its own continuance. I see it riffling among other potentially antagonizing memories, working to get me engaged so I will stoke the flames anew. Provoked anger is more than roiling energy, it's a hunger.

My partner wakes slowly, thankfully. I am calm and self-possessed by the time she surfaces. It is late in the morning, but breakfast can wait. In fact, today, it's better that it does.

When my lover has gone away again, her home, her job, I write her of desire:

She explains anorexia to me, wide scars grown old

Radiant heat brushing from everything in her touching

Under streaks of pink, she says inner forces of will

and domination of the body

and opposing exhibitionist influence

something to parade the child's bones under Walnut Ave's

chinquapin oaks

the patriotic music from the bandstand.

And she sleeps.

Explaining what remains, my cheeks flush, a day of

sunshine, on a highway proposing

that we are one.

I was asleep before we reentered the highway with two new

sources of refined sugar

Both for me: To stay awake, my hands on the wheel like I

grip her arm

as a thousand tail lights inhale before us like a wall rising

from black water.

"Did you eat the peanut butter cup?" she will ask me the
next day
"The cranberry juice? I can't remember."
And I'll stroke her arm in the white bed
to reach for its fire
silence the TV bolted behind me from a switch at her side.

An illuminated breath
A green quiet line.

The reflection of myself in a $4 pair of glasses says I
am alive, behind a thousand closed doors
beneath a thousand severed cables, interrupted and
confiscated, the shipment of questionable material I've read
and wondered. Jailbroke my brain. Listen for the sound of
her exhaling. And breathe, I suppose.

"My heart can't swim," I say.
"The ocean is on fire," she says.
I beat my thigh

the roll of a match head

extinguishing itself as it falls.

And she sleeps.

Someone else's finger traces the buttons of her spine

I'm swallowing the sea, compacted, completed

by the absolute absence

that comes as suddenly as the next wave

for a child running in sandy shorts with a small blur on a

leash who notices only sunshine

exploding in every bead of water spiraling and streaking and

singing

in every possible direction

everything at once

like rapture.

Beyond the Epidemic

Normal sadness is to depression what normal growth is to cancer.

— Lewis Wolpert, *The Balance Within*

My answer befuddles my ex-wife. Wasn't the one she was expecting. "I'm doing good," I say during my first week into the treatment. "About seventy percent of the day."

Talking into the phone as I drive back from the nature park where I've been letting the two dogs — my support group — run in the wind and sun. "And you're off your Klonopin?" she asks incredulously.

Yeah, it strikes me, settling in.

"Why do you think that is?" she asks.

Why hasn't that steady round of panic attacks and suicidal depression followed the subtraction of my lithium, Wellbutrin, Prozac, and Klonopin? Why hasn't the me of summer 2012 returned as I'd been expecting?

Back then, she was the one who reminded me about the power of pills. She gave me permission, so to speak, to return to them after I'd been swamped by that tsunami of anxiety and depression. It would take nearly three months to get into a shrink for a prescription. In the meantime, I ground my teeth through a dozen panic attacks a day and reverberating suicidal urges. By the time I got my tube of little yellow tablets I had totally forgotten how strong and fast a good dose of Klonopin could be. And I had forgotten how much better being a little stoned at a work could make a meeting. I still shuttered myself at home after hours, however, and clawed the floors and walls begging relief. Begging, as my most recent therapist had encouraged me, for information about the root of my illness. It would prove to be worse than futile.

If I've ever come to believe with certainty that there is absolutely nothing but what we think there is, it was during this time. No matter how I twisted myself or amplified my hurt, nothing responded. Nothing appeared. It was Nothing that wrapped itself around me and offered me to myself.

Of course, my case was far from unique. These days, depression touches everything. It is the leading cause of disability worldwide in terms of lost work, draining the U.S. economy of an estimated $36.6 billion per year. By 2030, the World Health Organization expects depression to be the most damaging illness – socially and economically – in upper-income countries, outdone only by HIV/AIDS and early childhood mortality elsewhere.

Despite these epidemic numbers, cultural stigmas surrounding mental illness and the lack of resources allocated to assist the suffering mean as many as half of the afflicted never receive treatment for their conditions in this country, according to the WHO. In a report released on World Mental Health Day, October 10, 2012, UN Secretary-General Ban Ki-moon took the opportunity to call for a more honest and open dialogue about depression, what he called an "under-appreciated global health crisis." It's strange to think that an epidemic estimated to impact 350 million people around the globe still needs defining. There should be no mysteries, no surprises surrounding any "global health crisis."

Biologist, author, and former depression-sufferer Lewis Wolpert struggled to give the illness its due by naming his 1999 work *Malignant Sadness* to "emphasize the very serious nature of a depressive illness and also to reflect my conviction that normal sadness is to depression what normal growth is to cancer. "Severe depression borders on being beyond description," he continues. "It is a quite different state, a state that bears only a tangential resemblance to normal emotion." Symptoms include a scattershot of maladies such as sadness, numbness, dullness, apathy, suicidal thoughts, crying spells, irritability, anger, insomnia, lethargy, fatigue, hallucinations, delusions, difficulty concentrating or making decisions, hopelessness, loss of self-esteem, anxiety, hypochondria, loss of interest, inability to feel pleasure, and on, and on.

But perhaps the strangest thing about depression is that despite hundreds of millions of dollars sunk into research and treatment over the years, and the seeming discovery of one miraculous drug after another, mental illness in America is still booming. While the number of adults in the United States on disability due to mental illness has climbed from roughly 500,000 in 1950 to 1.25 million in 1987 to 3.97 million in 2007, the real tumult is happening among those still transitioning into the workplace.

A 2008 report of the U.S. General Accounting Office reported that one of every 16 young adults – or 2.4 million – between 18 and 26 had a "serious" mental illness in 2006. And even that figure is likely to be greater than reported, since the incarcerated, institutionalized, and homeless – populations known to harbor high numbers of mentally ill – were not counted in the study.

Either there is something in the metaphorical water or there is a serious problem with the way mental illness is diagnosed and treated. Or both.

Into the Leech Tree

It seemed to her that there were seven wood-brown birds flying
through the forest, and then suddenly one of them turned white
and fell down dead.

— William T. Vollman, *The Ice Shirt*

At one end of the building in yet another sterile hospital hallway a woman lay twitching on the floor. Her head was to the side, her eyes closed. Above her a man in a blue jumpsuit, hard hat, and dustpan was standing like a barricade. A woman in a suit peeked out of a side door. "Did anyone call anyone?" she asked.

I walked around the quivering body, between the blue man and the bouncing head, seeking out a small cafe cut into a recess in the wall, and sat down with two small plastic cups of fruit. I checked my computer.

I checked the time. Five minutes until my session.

A team of paramedics came rolling a tall stretcher and two bags of gear toward the inconvenient convulsion. Before passing slowly around the corner, one towheaded medic asked the others in a nasally syrup-drenched drawl, "Wa'appened? Did she fain' when they tol' her how much her beel wuz?"

I typed in a few notes, closed my computer, and bussed my table. The trio came rolling from the other direction, returning with their empty crash cart.

Upstairs the Eggbeater, as I've come to call the sTMS machine (optimistically registered as the "NEST," or NeoSync-EEG Synchronized TMS), danced on my head. It wobbled, I think, like a quarter-greedy Nevada motel bed. I thought about all the weeks of treatment ahead of me and how to plan some fun weekend time with my partner, her child, and my daughter. I imagined kayaks and how I would fasten them to my roof if I had them. I thought my daughter may like her own craft. Imagined floating the group into a field of familiar low-hanging, litter-filtering branches we know as the Llano River Leech Tree.

I opened my eyes and almost laughed out loud. We'd floated into the leech tree again.

Overmedicating

Emotions are what we live and die for. Diseases are what we die from.

— Esther Sternberg, *The Balance Within*

What lies behind this depression epidemic is the million-dollar question. Like the coalition of forces fingered in the collapse of global honeybee populations, depression culprits are everywhere and definitive answers nowhere. Exposure to environmental toxins is known to contribute to mental illness. As are food allergies, inflammation, and the Standard American Diet. The role of bacteria, inherited genetics, trauma, and substance abuse are also understood to play a role, and research continues into possible contributions made by electromagnetic radiation emitted by power lines, cell phone towers, and Wi-Fi networks.

However, as psychiatry's bible, the *Diagnostic and Statistical Manual of Mental Disorders*, has continued to widen the definitions of who should be considered sick, the medical response has narrowed. Psychiatric drugs have become the first – and frequently the only – prescription offered by psychiatrists. While my now dismissed pharmaceutical cocktail likely helped save my life, in our quick-fix culture many don't even take the time to consult a psychiatrist before popping their pills. Instead, they hit up the family doctor with specific Google-informed drug requests.

"I see lots of people who get put on anti-depressants and anti-anxiety medications a couple days after a death in the family, by their primary care docs," Austin-based psychiatrist Dr. William M. Konyecsni tells me. "Well, feeling sad after a death is normal. I've also had parents give their kids their medication and they don't think twice about it, and we're talking things like Klonopin and Xanax. I mean, we have to experience and feel things to learn and grow. Not all of it is bad." These powerful chemicals change the way people's brains work, even those without the diagnoses that are presumed to have preceded their use. Some have begun to challenge the long-term implications of that practice.

"In the last 30 years, we've greatly expanded the boundaries – or psychiatry has – of what is considered ill. More people are getting treated, too. From a societal point of view you want to ask: Is that a good thing?" author Robert Whitaker said. "Are they better off five years later, 10 years later? ... Are they in less psychological distress? Unfortunately, the evidence it just not there."

Whitaker, an investigative journalist-turned-burr under the saddle of Big Pharma, insists in his most recent book, *Anatomy of an Epidemic: Magic Bullets, Psychiatric Drugs, and the Astonishing Rise of Mental Illness in America*, that the long-term outcome is actually worse for those placed on psychiatric drugs than for those who go without. Though his work has historically stressed the troubling history of antipsychotics and schizophrenia, *Anatomy* unearths numerous case studies that show similar patterns at work in the popular treatment of anxiety, depression, and bipolar disorder. "There's pretty good evidence that the drugs increase the chronicity of the disorder in the aggregate. That does not mean nobody is doing well on the drugs. People are. It's just that it doesn't improve their recovery rates [in the long-term]; it actually worsens their recovery rates."

It's another reminder that I have to take charge of my illness—regular exercise, meditation, yoga, vitamins and "nutraceuticals." I've even begun to research buying my own field-pulsing magnetic device for after the trial's conclusion.

The Unsung

The totality of life is merely a fancy kind of rust.

— H.J Muller, *Life*

There are so many books around me, speaking of the tombs of writers and heroes, of destiny, invasion, famine, invention. Implied in each but addressed in none is the unknowable weight of human muscle, of faceless labor, and unremarked eons of evolutionary effort — the billions who never secured a pen scratch of recognition, a name on vellum or papyrus.

The backyard chimes. I hear them buffeted by the breeze. Like the ring on my finger, they'll outlive me. I'll stop hearing one day. But the chimes?

I'm reminded of expectations. The ones we're raised on. The manipulating myths of a child's infinite abilities and society's accommodating elasticity ever making room for them as they grow. Damnable stuff. And the silence now of the chimes followed by a rapid return of their dancing scale, out of sequence and again brief. The dog at my feet swallows a snore, shakes and stretches, relaxing into her crescent mold in the carpet.

With or without us, things somehow resolve.

Smiling Inside

*Behold, I am sending you out as sheep in the midst of wolves, so
be wise as serpents and innocent as doves.*

— Matthew 10:16, *The Holy Bible*

The morning smells like something you want to stuff
your pockets full of. An early morning shower has
provided for the magical mingling of earth and water,
followed by the stirring of birdsong. Now the sun
cutting sideways across the oak-dense scrub delivers the
necessary heat for an exhalation and stirring of winds.

Earth, water, air, and fire. Something higher?
Something the senses know but that the mind can't
recognize? (Would the tongue even be able to
pronounce it?) I'm sensing something deep in the
brambles with a taste for flesh. Something that would
like to be left alone with one of our dogs — *Just for a*

few minutes, I imagine the lip-curling request — but won't approach me. The food web here ends at my pair of weathered hiking boots. That fact makes the bundle of brooding blood-lust in the brush endearing, like a Build-A-Bear rocking in the woods. Furry creatures a la Jim Henson.

The only monsters to fear are the disgruntled and vengeful among my own kind and the tools they manufacture. My predecessors saw to that, stamping out the black bear and grizzly (*horribilis*, according to Linnaeus). The jaguar, cougar, red wolf. Before that, the short-faced bear, American cheetah, scimitar cat. It's to my benefit, but still I root for the coyotes, the red fox, horned owl, the hanger-on predators of this city.

To know that a hunt and feasting lives on, the continuing condensation of the many into the bodies of the few—once-warm and blood-rich beings woven into another's muscle and fat and bone. As removed as I am, standing here smelling the air, two dogs on retractable leashes and a plastic bag to collect their stool, I still know that I come from that. And I hunger.

Then it strikes me, these things I am able to consider only because I woke up smiling inside. How did that happen?

Sure, I'm enamored of my new bike that carries me to the train and back each day. These two still-uneaten dogs who pile up so nicely with my parents' silent scampering mop of a dog when the temperature dips outside. The rampantly pearling fabric of my Swazi-produced sweater guarding me from the gusts of grey cold. I wouldn't have recognized any of these pleasures if there hadn't first been a peacefulness, a contentedness.

It's an emotional settling I've observed more and more recently. I've been monitoring my emotions like a lab tech on a suspect pulse for so long now, steering myself again and again around the edges of explosive anger and disappointment. Refusing to be sucked down, I've clung to the sheltering coast of what I hoped was well-being. And, now, I appear to have arrived, to have surfaced. Weigh anchor.

Strange as it feels to say, I am happy.

With the gloom and fear momentarily at bay, it's worth commenting on something else I notice. In this mind, this happy mind, there is a near-total absence of self regard. That mirror that is so often fastened before my face forcing me to observe myself through every other person's point of view — disapproving ones, universally — has fallen. My own inner critic is silent, too. I find I am lighter, less central, more fluid in the world because of it. It's an interesting sensation, this very natural sinking into the fabric and movement of living.

Interruption

At the most basic level, everything is for sale and everything is an exchange.

— Former Eli Lilly drug rep Shahram Ahari, *Unhinged: The Trouble With Psychiatry*

The principal investigator, the big dog, interrupts my 30-minute session mid-way to introduce himself. Shake hands. Thank me for participating. I'm trying to focus my eyes in the low light while my thoughts meander like dandelion fluff.

He tells me (apropos of what?) that NeoSync didn't want to offer participants who got the placebo, the intentionally broken machine, a free round of so-called "open label" treatment after the initial six-week study. I'm only mildly surprised when he tells me that he pushed back and got them to relent. I don't have an opportunity to tell him that without that guarantee I wouldn't have signed up. It's not like we're getting paid to put our brains beneath this hardware. Had I the clarity required of the moment, I probably would have added how strange it felt to be interrupted in the near dark, a shadowy figure looming over my reclined body.

I want to get back to the rattling of a possibly dysfunctional machine, to thoughts of my new bicycle. But he wants to tell me how excited he is about sTMS. To say that adverse outcomes are so unlikely that he submitted himself to a session. "He did," the fashion-plate facilitator says as if I would have any reason to doubt. "I have a picture of it."

When I'm finally allowed to return to my session, I imagine my gray matter swelling upward like the ocean drawn by moon-force desire. I imagine my neurons stretching like a trellis-ensconced lover reaching out an arm for his lover's balcony lip.

"Thirteen minutes to go," the facilitator interrupts.

I have to start again. There isn't enough time.

Rebooting the Brain

Look out! The first is pestiferous, the second mortiferous.
  — First recipient of electroshock therapy, 1938

"Look out!" the Italian man bellowed indeed, presumably first spitting the rubber tube out of his mouth meant to keep him from biting into his tongue. The 80 volts was merely "pestiferous," or annoying, he said. But this second jolt of 90 volts he called "deadly" as he sprung into a sitting position on the operating table.

It was the third shock, delivered to the man suffering what sounds like a bout of severe paranoia through electrodes wired to the head. The first recipient of what came to be called "electroshock," more recently electroconvulsive therapy, or ECT, received another 11 treatments before being discharged hallucination-free.

Ugo Cerletti got the idea for electrifying patients while viewing pigs being rendered unconscious by 125 volts of electricity prior to their dismemberment at a slaughterhouse. He didn't stick solely to the electric side of the equation, either.

From Wikipedia:

> "Cerletti called his treatment 'electroshock' and developed a theory that it worked by causing the brain to produce vital substances that he called 'acro-agonines' (from the Greek for 'extreme struggle'). He put his theory into practice by injecting patients with a suspension of electroshocked pig brain, with encouraging results. Electroshocked pig brain therapy was used by a few psychiatrists in Italy, France and Brazil but did not become as popular as ECT."

I can't imagine.

In humans, the electrification was intended to be beneficial, to inspire a mood-cleansing seizure. Of course it took some time to get it right. Many have suffered deeply. The technology has changed considerably over the years however and today electroconvulsive therapy is frequently the first choice of doctors for patients with depressive disorders that are resistant to drug therapy. One continuing side effect of the technology, however, plagues the treatment: loss of memory.

How does ECT work? There are theories, but as

Daniel Carlat writes in *Unhinged: The Trouble With Psychiatry:* "[t]he major problem with ECT is identical to the problem with psychiatric medication. ... While ECT works, we have no idea how or why."

Calling it a "safe well-studied medical procedure," Dr. James Potash wrote something of a majority opinion for the psychiatric establishment in an ABC News essay. ECT, he writes, "seems to reboot the emotional machinery of the brain, in the same way that pressing Ctrl-Alt-Delete on the computer can sometimes provide a fresh start when the digital computer brain is stuck."

Now "rebooting" is a term this generation can grasp. It's the same terminology I heard when I first inquired about TMS. "We don't really know how it works," one TMS coordinator told me. "But we think it sort of stimulates the neurons. In a lot of severely depressed patients this area of the brain has very low activity. We think TMS can 'reboot' the brain and get those neurons active again."

I have to admit. I liked what I heard. In fact, I used it multiple times when explaining to my closest friends and family what I intended to do: reboot.

After twelve sessions, I've caught nerves in my face twitching hours after treatments. I'm not falling asleep easily at night either. That's been going on a week now. The downside of an upside, perhaps? I noticed something else unexpected, an energy to make, to do.

A Palpable Buzzing

There was a running interest in what effects people's standing in the field of radio energy have ... if you could hypnotize somebody easier if he was standing in a radio beam.

— MKULTRA Director Sidney Gottlieb

Something is happening.

Week one of my clinical trial was utter discouragement. The machine's Playskool racket coupled with a depressive crash told me I'd gotten the placebo. I was that unlucky bastard randomly consigned to six weeks of wasted time.

In week two I was keen to credit what improvements I saw to the strengths of my own healing commitment. I was simply willing myself to rebound. I'd changed my life in so many ways that improvement was to be expected. The move into my parents' house with its decreased responsibilities, as many naps as I needed, no fear of having to explain to old acquaintances what I'd been up to these three months post work. I thought favorably of the new bicycle and my exponential increase in exercise and clean air, sunshine. I did that.

But a four-day migraine followed by nights of sleeping trouble has me reassessing. The headache alone, the sleeplessness alone, but combined? That screams side effects. And that means someone left my machine turned on.

Two in the morning and there was a palpable buzzing in my body. A latent energy I could feel lying in the dark. It moved in circles in a kind of mist showing no signs of slowing. It's the same energy that had kept me up working past midnight. It would piss me off if not for the fact that the new energy brought an ability to be interested in the world. I was up late because I wanted to be, because I'm engaging, reading and writing. There was something to be done.

Both the trouble sleeping and the new levels of passion and acuity informing my nocturnal scribblings were unusual. Even in healthier times I rarely stayed into the early morning working. I mean, hate to admit it, but I've always been a slut for sleep.

So I was suspicious when I got on the train this morning and cracked my book, *The Body Electric: Electromagnetism and the Foundation of Life*. Almost immediately I read a passage about a 1930's Russian study on one particular therapeutic use for low-level electricity.

Russian doctors claimed their "elektroson" technique, which used electrodes on the eyelids and behind the ears to deliver weak electric currents pulsing at calming brain-wave frequencies, could impart the benefits of a full night's sleep in two to three hours. And what exactly is "weak electric currents pulsing at calmative brain-wave frequencies" if not sTMS? While few scientists in the States publicly pursued an interest in electromagnetism in the biological sciences after the 1920s, the Russians pressed on.

Here and in much of the rest of the world researchers were too sickened by the abuses perpetrated by the electrotherapy contingent in the eighteenth and nineteenth centuries, Robert Becker writes, to move deeper into such research. A veritable body blow was delivered by Abraham Flexner, who in a major evaluation of American medicine in 1910 "denounced the clinical use of electric shocks and currents, which had been applied, often over-enthusiastically, to many diseases since the mid-1700s. Electrotherapy sometimes seemed to work, but no one knew why, and it had gotten a bad name from the many charlatans who'd exploited it."

With the breakthrough discovery of penicillin and quickening of biochemical knowledge, the playing field belonged "almost exclusively" to the chemical approach to illness. A hard winter set in on those interested in the electrical nature of life. Consider the sTMS trial I'm taking part in a sort of Western rebound.

When I mentioned all this to the facilitator, she offered that herbal teas may help with the insomnia. But when I pressed, she allowed that, yes, headaches and insomnia are frequently reported side effects of sTMS treatment. So now I know. Or I think I know. We're chasing the Russians.

Anti-Christ

Anger has become your friend—it helps you maintain some
semblance of control.

— Peter A. Levine, *Walking the Tiger: Healing Trauma*

Standing at the corner in an old green army jacket.
Big plastic olive buttons, double-stitched eyelets, and a
flaking white upside-down cross on a sharp-cut-but-
fraying lapel. I'm approached by someone. Man?
Woman? They point to St. Peter's cross, the product of
an adolescent's anger and a bottle of White-Out, that
old typewriting correction fluid all but eradicated by
the Information Revolution.
     "Does that mean you're a … a … "
Does that mean I'm a what?
     It's been a week since the dream, this sliver only
coming to mind at a stop light on the way to my train

this morning. I know the jacket as the one I wore when I was thirteen. I replaced it later with a jean jacket that I decorated with metal spikes and markers. On the back I reproduced the lengthy liner notes (a veritable manifesto) from the hardcore punk compilation "Rat Music for Rat People" LP.

Does that mean I'm a what? An antichrist?

Granted a religious rebellion is a perfect fit for this country, "One Nation Under God" inserted into the Pledge during the Red Scare. I can see a value in that. But even with the symbol on my breast I'm not sure I would have ever considered myself anti-Christ. Or maybe I did. There was that short season where I jumped the tracks, that biting season during which one goes from being a child of others, a product of culture and upbringing, to being a self-orientated individual living in response to those forces and their own inner music.

Abandoning my Christian upbringing would have made sense, possibly a very necessary rebellion, in the search for self. Though, to be honest, it was also likely a rabid conformity to a new master, punk rock. Anti-hypocrisy. Anti-intolerance. Anti-religion. Anti-racism. Anti-consumerism. Anti-war. Even anti-Christian. (These notoriously weak exemplars of their savior need an organized resistance to keep them from getting flabby, after all.) All these contrary positions remained as my rejection of church and God softened with time and suffering.

Depression, cutting, panic attacks, an exhausting anger, and drug and alcohol overdoses were great tenderizers. Increasingly I found myself wanting the embrace of Sunday School religion, to hear the sound of my mother playing good Methodist hymns on the piano, something soft, safe, loving. I'd seen enough by seventeen to know evil was strong in the world and yet I was ashamed of what I wanted.

I read a paperback New Testament — one with those stick figure illustrations — secretly at night. It took time. But when conversion finally came it was a fundamentalist whirlwind that would remake me to the core, repositioning me in the cultural and political and social landscape in ways I couldn't understand at the time. It was bona fide born-again experience that flooded my being with a revelatory acceptance and love on one hand and new rules, definitions, and cultural struggles — in some cases, outright fabrications — on the other.

All would be knit into my faith as a single thread, making for a messy divorce three years later, and an abiding dissatisfaction today, a quarter-century on. That's how long its been since I have been able to hold my arms up in a congregation and profess my love for a unified deity. Honestly, I miss the intimacy. Holding hands with near strangers, head bowed in prayer. I could go on.

It's not just the lapel embellishment that brings it all to mind now. Honestly, the questions bound up in those few years are never far from my mind. The monotheist's mysterious god of a thirsty much-contested geography accentuated later by a babe in a manger or an epileptic in a cave, depending on whom

you ask, lives on my train. Or perhaps in one of the
homeless tents tucked away among the fragments of
countryside between stops. (After the cement batching
plant and the natural gas compressor station?)

In any event, His folks are on high alert. It seems
hardly an engagement transpires on the tracks in
which He isn't dragged into it.

God and Weed

In times of war, we pray for victory and we believe, or hope, that God is on our side.

— Andrew Newberg, *Born to Believe*

He's fifty, give or take. Wearing those wraparound sunglasses that create an ocular unibrow. Straight-up redneck and poet. "I write lyrics and poems," he volunteered. "I even had one of my poems published."

He rattled off a good thirty consistently rhymed lines about coming from a long line of men "who did what's right," about taking his shotgun and "good dog 'Red' " to "cross the sands, looking for the leader of the Taliban."

Brave. True. Black. White.

On conclusion, he popped his hand up for a high five. I high-fived him. He offered his fist lower down for a fist bump. I fist-bumped him. They say to never wake a sleepwalker.

He said God had probably introduced us for a reason. I'm skeptical. Last week it was a fellow suggesting I read Psalms for my depression, departing with a satisfied smile after I'd let him explain why we should reinstitute the gold standard.

But I don't know, my dude could be right. As we talk I learned he too has a history of depression, anxiety, schizophrenia. But he won't take meds. They messed him up good back in the day, he said. And, yeah, he's interested in this sTMS study I'm doing. It could be for him. I rattled off prerequisites. You can't have a history of substance abuse in the last twelve months, for instance. My Very Clean-cut Redneck snorted. He went on about his philosophy of pills and illness. But I wanted to know how he gets by when things get bad? He admitted things still get bad.

His lips folded down as a single finger pointed up as if he's prepared to say something about cutting down the cherry tree. "God," he says.

A pause.

He angled his cup toward me with a smile. "And beer." Both he and his lady friend carry the over-sized plastic cups.

Another pause.

He leaned in and lowered his goggles to show me his eyes. "You really want to know? You want to know the truth?

"Weed," he said. "Weed."

His meter and delivery were immaculate. My

poetry-loving heart gave him another very high five.

Cortex on Sunspots

*We are blind to more than 99.999 percent of the light that
actually exists in the universe.*

— Gary E. Schwartz

I'm coming to realize that before I ever contacted
the sTMS study's facilitator about the trial I was
receiving electromagnetic "therapy" from our star, our
moon, the earth, and a thousand and one devices
dreamed up to shrink our planet. As a planter painted
by my partner in honor of my trial participation with
silver loops embracing a blue and green planet, ours is
a magnetic world full of invisible forces not only
moving through us but moving us.

Your brain. On sunspots.

Our inverted bowls of bone may protect the squishy
space upstairs from bumps and falls, but it offers little

resistance to solar winds, the electromagnetic fields of power poles and sub-power stations, or even the subtle vibrations of the Chromebook into which I type these words. In fact, researchers are beginning to link the sunspot activity that disrupts our natural geomagnetic field with health impacts, including increased rates of psychotic behavior and institutionalization.

Michael Persinger, a researcher at the Consciousness Research Lab at Laurentian University, found a correlation between thirty-seven years of haunting reports and recorded geomagnetic activity, according to Mary Roach writing in *Spook: Science Tackles The Afterlife.* Persinger published his findings in *Neuroscience Letters* in 1998, Roach writes, adding:

"In a similar study three years later, University of Iowa psychologists Walter and Steffani Randall examined monthly fluctuations in solar winds (which influence the earth's geomagnetics) to see if they mirrored monthly ups and downs in 'humanoid hallucinations' culled from old Society of Psychical Research records. Indeed, both showed peaks in April and September with a trough in between."

Persinger has moved on to reproduce otherworldly experiences in a laboratory setting in research subjects by using electromagnetic fields. Plainly, he's made them see "synthetic ghosts." The author put herself through the ordeal and reported seeing faces and hearing a "a police car in the distance," despite being in a sound-proofed room.

Persinger explains this phenomena by pointing out that people exposed to high levels of electromagnetic frequency have lower levels of the anti-convulsive melatonin, leaving them prone to "micro-seizures" and the resulting hallucinations this can lead to. I know I've had my share of such. Many I've been able to explain in a way that worked for me. Others, not so much.

My trio of magnets sing again tomorrow. I'm thinking maybe they're doing more than picking a fight with my depression. This could be the reboot that so many others have promised before.

'3,000 Pulses'

That is all I want in life: for this pain to seem purposeful.

— Elizabeth Wurtzel, *Prozac Nation*

Martha Rhodes first received TMS treatment in 2010. Like me, the former NYC ad exec had suffered for decades, done poorly on a range of pharmaceuticals, and shied away from ECT. She was desperate for something outside psychiatry's traditional toolbox when her sister faxed her a full-page ad from *Connecticut Magazine* trumpeting the "newest technology to treat depression without discomfort or drugs."

For Rhodes, TMS took three weeks to start pulling her out of her death-wish depression, and that followed a dangerous mood dip in week two. "Your brain is being reconnoitered," the author of *3,000 Pulses: Surviving Depression with TMS* and *3,000 Pulses*

Later: A Memoir of Surviving Depression Without Medication
told me. "You could experience happiness, then
sadness, then happiness again. It takes, I'm going to
say, a good 20 visits."

In my dim room, I drifted through multiple levels of
awareness as the Egg did its thing in the fourth week of
the trial. Out of the darkness and the day's troubled
thoughts I felt a moth fluttering against my right ear
and cheek. Would I break protocol if I swiped after it?
Opened my eyes? I mentally tracked the fluttering for
what felt like minutes. Velvet wings brushed against
the invisible hairs above the earlobe, almost
imperceptible insect steps moved along the ear's ridge
before the fluttering sensation resumed again. It
dawned on me that the likelihood a moth was
haunting the research hospital testing room was
probably low.

Were these nerves activating? I watched again and
observed a slender pain move through the inside of my
cheek. Felt another energetic tentacle spread behind
my eye. If the electrical stimuli around my head and
face suggested I was not getting the placebo treatment,
a coexistent surge of sadness—brought on by a recent
letter denying me health insurance due to my mental-
health history—also meant that even a cutting-edge
depression-buster wasn't an automatic happy pill.

In those first weeks, I'd gone through days of high
agitation, suffered a multi-day migraine, and started
having trouble sleeping—all things the attending
doctor warned I could experience. But I'd also
discovered new-found physical energy and a

noticeably sharpened mental acuity that allowed me to steam through book after book on psychology, psychiatry, electromagnetism, religion, and shamanism.

"The stuff is happening," I wrote at the time. "I'm sure it's the device."

Doing, Doing

Fly in the buttermilk, Shoo, fly, shoo.

  – "Skip to My Lou," children's song

    A sharp adult whistle reverberating in the tight tiled space of the hospital bathroom suggests "Skip, Skip, Skip To My Lou." A child's voice begins singing the nursery rhyme, chirping merrily in Mandarin or possibly Korean, I think. The man I take for the father prompts, "Anchisaurus!" and the child obediently starts in on a new melody about (I imagine) the misadventures of an adorable baby-sized dino with razor-sharp leaf-shredding teeth. Then again I don't speak Korean.

    It's all so resoundingly happy out there. There joy in my poop stall as well. The weekly assessment confirms my self-assessment: "Happy."

It's my fourth assessment since the start of the trial and my sleep has returned to normal. I'm irritable and anxious and worried at times (just as anyone, I suspect). Sex drive normal. Hunger normal. I see myself as no better or worse than others I respect. Normal again. Don't obsess or count repeatedly. And I both dream at night and plan for a future during the day. No thoughts of self-harm. No suicidal nothing. Normal the battery of questions leads me to believe.

During a tiring weekend with all the family familiarly navigating perceived slights and exclusions, I was able to recognize my sensitivities as (mostly) fallacious constructions and adjust my behavior appropriately. I'm participating in and enjoying family times together, while winnowing out the potential emotional pitfalls. All these positives, they come from one place—a brain waking up, retuned.

I kept remembering a line from some promotional literature about TMS. The magnetic pulses of TMS are believed to combat depression (as well as Parkinson's and coma and other states of diminished brain function) by "exciting" the neurons. Like at a party. Consider my neurons flooded in confetti and jubilantly discarded wrapping paper. I was writing like crazy. When not writing, I'm reading. When not reading, I was riding my bicycle. When not riding my bicycle, I was doing my laundry, paying my bills, washing my dogs. And when I wasn't doing any of that, I was thinking why not. Been asleep for so long, so much to do.

I felt solid, embodied in a way I haven't in a long

time. I don't know how else to describe it, but I felt
connected within myself, a fully integrated, highly
functioning system: a synergy. I guess it should come
as no surprise that I became utterly fascinated by the
process I was experiencing and desperate to
understand bioelectricity, electromagnetism, all the
invisible inputs and outputs underappreciated by
Western medicine, these emerging modes of healing.

Outside the bathroom a woman was mopping the
hall. I intuitively spread the bones in my feet like they
teach you in yoga class and place my shoes down
carefully. Flat step. Flat step. I was smiling. The
process was so natural, so smooth, so important. So
fun to walk when the sign warns that the floor is wet.

Everything again, I think.

Everything matters again.

Tangerine Dream

Feelings come and go like clouds in a windy sky. Conscious breathing is my anchor.

– Thich Nhat Hanh

It occurs to me that in all this narration I've given short shrift to the importance of mindfulness in my recovery. Before I ever found my way to sTMS, before I ever left my job a rattled embarrassed mess, I found Sara teaching at a privately owned South Texas psychiatric hospital.

There was a dozen of us in a room being lectured by this woman in those toed rubber shoes that look like something the Navy Seals dreamed up. Something for creeping sea-bottom maneuvers?

She joins her hands and bows slightly. "Namaste."

Her smile disarms.

"We love you Sara," sing-songs a hulking mass in the corner whose very teeth appear to have their own workout regimen.

"Catch!" Sara says, throwing a small orange to the quiet woman on my right. "Catch!" My turn. I'm far from happy, but work up a smile anyway. She smiles back. Or maybe she never stopped. I forgive her shoes in an instant, am refocused, present in her gaze. Are we having a moment? The light in her recognizing the light in me?

The toss-and-catch moves quickly around the circle.

If there is any self-discovery taking place at this treatment center it has to fit within these 35-minute sessions after lunch each day. I have yet to find anything more valuable here than the people suffering with me and Sara's instruction.

On Monday, she explains the many steps the mind makes between an unwelcome stimuli and a responding action. She suggests that unwelcome stimuli as someone cutting you off in traffic. One from the circle suggests one potential responding action to be tossing a flaming molotov cocktail into the offending vehicle's window. There's a lot of suicidal military here. Many careers redlined because they made the mistake of asking for help.

Group sessions are regularly divided between civilians and military, but it's not a hard division. Most days it's obvious the distance is artificial, our common struggles with mental illness a great leveler. Other times real difference surfaces, such as the day Ben explained casually how he would feel no sympathy if someone chose to break the law by walking outside of the crosswalk and was run over and killed. ("I'd help them," he insisted. "But I wouldn't feel sorry.")

On the day we're led through the tangerine meditation we hold the fruits in our hands and inspect them carefully, bounce them in our hands, hold them to the light. We explore their smells as we puncture the flesh, feel the spray against our skin, sugars turning sticky between our fingers. The shape, the texture, the taste. Sara's lured us into this centering moment before we even realize our high-revving fears and screaming internal protests have faded into the background. We've unseated our illnesses with tangerines.

If only they knew, religions around the world would quake at the news: Tangerines are the answer.

On Wednesday we're put with partners and instructed to quiz each other by repeating two questions over and over. "Who are you?" and "What do you want?" It's awkward at first. I'm scared to speak honestly about my hippier inclinations. I don't really want to hear about Ben's love affair with law and order.

"Who are you?" Ben asks, wiggling pen on paper.
A father.
"Who are you?"
A friend.
"Who are you?"
A boss. A son. A lover, partner.
"Who are you?"
A seeker. A writer. A hiker. A lover of nature.

I'm ashamed of my judgment of him when I see he shares many of these same identifications. He loves the outdoors, his family, his wife.

"What do you want?"

We want love.

"What do you want?"

We want to be good parents. To be true friends. To be helpful.

To know what's beyond this life, I say.

To go to heaven, he says.

In twenty minutes the exercise is over. We put our chairs back in place. Collect our things. He'll go to see the psychiatrist to discuss his meds; I'll go to physical therapy to play Battleship. We meet each other's eyes briefly on the way out, nod our recognitions with tight lips.

Namaste.

III. Awakening at Dusk

Meeting the Dragon

Dreaming is a powerful problem-solving mode of the brain — it is a doorway into the healing realm.

—Jonathan G. Zuess, *The Wisdom of Depression*

Reading *The Wisdom of Depression* about the power of dreams to heal psychological wounds, I'm reminded of dreams past.

One in particular, actually, from more than two decades ago.

In it I'm walking across a bombed-out city. All is shades of grey—no visible life anywhere. I stop and peer into a pile of rubble and sense something stirring within. A dragon moves into view, it's skin swirling in curling overlapping wisps of rainbow. I see a female join him, placing her left claw upon his back. We stare at each other for a long time. No words are spoken.

As my mental energy is being restored by daily magnetic treatments I've seen my comprehension ramping up. Hard academic books that were just too dense before begin to reveal themselves to me. But recognizing the relationships between my dreams and my woundedness, between the hopes and fears expressed in nightly narrative, is not always straightforward.

There is the dream of the kitchen in which I'm the chef of a new restaurant. We're preparing to open to the public but there are few victuals about. I struggle to make use of a few potatoes. A tomato. I do what I can on the cutting block, but what will happen when the customers arrive, I wonder. Eventually the orders come. I do my best to ship the dishes out quickly, but I forget crucial steps. The pasta noodles I forget to bake before I boil (or boil before I bake?) and they turn into blocks of undifferentiated slop on the plate. There is hardly enough marinara sauce. The diners are less than enthusiastic.

Gradually the kitchen fills with staff and there is foodstuff everywhere, but more problems follow. The tomatoes are hidden under baking sheets (pasta sauce plays something of a central role here). Pans are left on the stove to smolder and smoke. It's not clear the finished plates are any better when we're finished with them then when they were raw ingredients. Confusion.

Another night it's a dream of dolphins.

A large school of dolphins entering the mouth of

the Rio Grande from the Gulf, swimming northwest. They're dying off in huge numbers, converted to drifting gelatinous shapes in the water, nearly unidentifiable. There's a dozen or two out in front still, moving forward, deeper into the continent. There's a group of us watching, tracking them, getting ready to move into the brush. We're being taught to know the natural world. To better explain it for others.

There are dreams of ex bosses, ex partners. As I turn them around in my mind, I think I should be able to reintegrate the dragon dream from so long ago, accept it in the seemingly generous spirit it was intended. Could be it can help me integrate so many seemingly oppositional beliefs--my valuing of satanic-rebel wisdom, respect for the disobedience that brought us fire and knowledge of opposites, my obsessions over sacrifice, compassion, and eternal love.

As if summoned, the dragon returned last night.

I'm in a bookstore with a Tibetan man on a speaking tour. Thinking of the spiritual leaders who guided a Buddhist sangha I once attended, I tell the man I have Tibetan friends. He asks who they are but I can't remember any names, only that some had relocated to northern India. His partner, who I take to be the subject of the speaking tour shows up. He's very tall, very strong. I'm getting ready to ship my bike back to Tibet with them so a friend can use it for her travels. She and I discuss how much to insure it for and decide on $300.

Then I'm outside looking across the highway. I see a dull black tube descending from the sky, extending from its middle like an unraveling tube of tar paper. As the funnel forms I see there are different bands of bright color peeking through the opening gaps. I get my camera phone ready and start taking video as the ever-expanding tube starts bouncing across the sky in huge black rolls filled with luminous primary colors. I wonder if it is bringing destruction on the ground. Looking closer I see a car getting swept up on the outer edge of a roll, but somehow the vehicle has a burning effect on the funnel and forces a retreat.

I wake. I make notes. I fall asleep again and dream something that leaves me smiling though I don't recall what for after my mother hollers out that I have overslept. It is time to get to the train.

My dulled mind didn't recognize the dragon in that tube of tar paper until after I had written it all down.

Betrayal

*To speak of happy accident is not to deny the negative side of
chance.*

— Lewis Hyde, *Trickster Makes This World*

As I round up on my sixth and final week of sTMS
treatment, I have come to finally understand the
critical link between energy and depression.
Depression is not just despondency or self-loathing or
overwhelming crippling sadness. I understand now
with my energy returning that my lifting depression is
not a banishment of unhappiness or disappointment or
frustration, key players in my depressed experience. All
those things are still here, but the vital energy
expressed in my body and new mental clarity allow me
to to work around those feelings. It gives me the
strength to work with them as partners instead of

crumbling before an overpowering force.

My likes and dislikes remain as they were before my last collapse, and I'm happy to report that observing dung beetles is as pleasurable as ever. It's welcome news. There were many times in the depths of the Great Bleakness that I honestly didn't know myself any more. I'd been fractured into these extreme personalities that seemed to have no conception of or compassion for one another. But as deep as I went, I see now that I wasn't lost. I was just forgotten for a time.

The facilitator says she is going to work with me to find an affordable therapist back in my home town. She floats the idea after my weekly assessment, which she says shows a downturn in mood.

Apparently "lots" of trial participants are showing the need for therapy (many for the first time, she adds) after getting sTMS treatment — "because they have all these new emotions bubbling up," she says, waggling her fingers in the air. "Drugs and this [gesturing to the Eggbeater] can't do everything."

What comes next is definitely not expected. I am told that there are indeed four weeks of "off-label" treatment available for those who received the sham or saw no improvement as stated in the agreement I had signed onto. However, I'm told now that those weeks can only be parceled out one week at a time—and only after one has demonstrated they are sick enough to deserve them.

Entering the trial, I expressed concern about the crapshoot nature of blind trials only to be told the study was designed to give me a two-out-of-three shot at a working machine. Instead it was a 50-50 chance, as the release of the study results in 2015 showed.

Still, I was determined to get the real stuff. I was going to get what I came for. Confidentially sharing my feelings about this bait-and-switch, the facilitator offers a little coaching. Don't lie, she says. Simply emphasize the difficult emotions I'm still experiencing and be more reserved when recounting the good ones. I plan to be good and sick on Monday. I've decided to game the system for all the certified therapy I can get.

Black Is Not Bleak

We are, each of us, as dark as Ramses' tomb. We are the black ink that fills the period at the end of the universe. We are cups of cosmic shadow.

— Gerald N. Callahan, *Faith, Madness, And Spontaneous Human Combustion*

In recounting my journey so far, I've certainly committed my share of errors. I'm sure I've failed to explain many nuances of the technologies explored. I've fallen down, certainly, as I've attempted to explain the depressed experience. And I've relied on tired language, repeating at least once the ill-advised use of the adjective "black" for all manner of sorry and malevolent states of being. The truth is, depressives are inheritors of Western culture's long denigration of blackness. If we accept that our melancholy temperaments are "black" in mood we also must wrestle with the meaning of blackness. Perhaps no other force did so much to shift indigenous concepts of blackness — the very color of our universe, of creation itself — as the colonial venture.

Racist terminology developed in tandem with and as justification for a race-based slave trade. This more-times-than-not religiously supported exploitation of life and labor is thought to have occurred somewhere between the conquest and enslavement of the Canary Islanders (where skin tones were not mentioned) and the wanton plundering of Africa.

In 1577, English navigator George Best blamed the color of black Africans, as was becoming popular in his day, on interpretations of Biblical genealogy. These "children of Ham" were said to be "still polluted with the same blot of infection," Scott Malcomson writes in "One Drop of Blood: The American Misadventure of Race."

Oh, sin.

By the time Christopher Columbus began bumping around the Caribbean, the encounters between the equally olive-complected natives and Spanish explorers were strangely cast in racial terms by the chroniclers who insisted the indigenous peoples were "amazed" by the Spaniards' "whiteness." Beards most likely amazed. The Spaniards' stench also. But their hue would have been very familiar.

Superstition about blackness in Western culture dates back to the Romans, but it took on new malevolence as the slave trade ramped up. Linguistic habits compounded these new cultural "truths." Evil deeds were "black as sin." Families had their "black sheep." Black days or moods were understood to be undesired. As all those who have experienced melancholy (as opposed to clinical depression or depression disorder) know — a "black" mood is frequently an intensely creative one. Melancholy, I've come to believe, is a deep state of problem-solving. The evil at work, if there is something thet qualifies for the term, is the absolute depletion of energy that allows antagonistic forces to play uncorrected. The paralyzing malaise prevents potentially restructuring insights from being tested and tried by application.

"Lincoln didn't do great work because he solved the problem of his melancholy," Joshua Wolf Shenk writes in "Lincoln's Melancholy: How Depression Challenged a President and Fueled His Greatness." "The problem of his melancholy was all the more fuel for the fire of his great work."

This color black — this powerful force that absorbs all colors and yet reflects none — has a noble history in human experience.

There's a Navajo creation story, for one, shared here as it is appears on the website First People.us:

The First World, Ni'hodilqil, was black as black wool. It had four corners, and over these appeared four clouds. These four clouds contained within themselves the elements of the First World. They were in color, black, white, blue, and yellow. The Black Cloud represented the Female Being or Substance. For as a child sleeps when being nursed, so life slept in the darkness of the Female Being. In this first world there were no people. There were beings known as the "Mist People" who had no form. They were the ones who would take form as all the biological creatures of this world. They were the potential of our biosphere. They were in the blackness of the Female Being.

Those of us who have been enfolded in the Substance know its power. It is the power of creation itself. Revel in your blackness.

Gospel Hospital

*Which of these two, God or the kamikazi, is the generator of the
other?*

— Régis Debray, *God: An Itinerary*

In my dream there was blood in my urine. Pissing
pink. My ex-wife takes me to the hospital. It's a
religiously based outfit with young volunteers. They
take a long time sorting out the line. When I get to the
front they want to pray with me for healing. I blow a
fuse. "I want to see the man with the knife," I shout.
More yelling follows.

We go to a second hospital. This one also turns out to
be religiously based, but in an African-American gospel
style. I find myself in a dense crowd of people willingly
bending my knees to pray.

Next, I'm in a cave that has been inhabited by a

coven gathered for ritual sacrifice. All around the top of the walls are what appear to be cross-shaped crystal lanterns, on one side they are positioned head down, on the other head up. The omniscient narrator explains the history of the cave, from Neolithic age up to its modern usage. Abducted people are brought here, people whose images are pasted on phone poles radiating out from their sites of capture. The woman exploring it with me is frustrated, angry, and scared. She is the last thing I see before I wake up.

On Fear

I am terrified by this dark thing/ That sleeps in me
— Sylvia Plath, *Ariel*

I'm afraid of being afraid and the onset of unbidden panic. Afraid of heights, violence, and embarrassment. I'm afraid of dying disappointed and of disappointing my parents. I'm afraid of depression, rage, and the various forces that take possession of my mind and body. Does admitting to the fears rob them of their power? If I admit to being afraid of being tortured or trapped underground? That I'll never be healthy enough to support myself again? That I'll never do those things I still dream of? In such hope, I continue my confession. I'm afraid I may have left the One True Faith. Of Hell. Of denying some vital aspect of who I am. That I may be a woman occupying a man's body (and the complications that would entail). Of making mistakes. Of being left alone. Being abandoned. Of being separated from love and of that separation lasting forever. Afraid of hurting my daughter's heart or her opinion of me. Of injuring those who have taken a risk by loving me. Afraid others will see how afraid I really am. Scared of dying before I've mastered each of the shapeshifts presented by this infinitely embracing and forgiving nature of reality. Afraid of being forgiven. Afraid of not being known. Afraid of not being complete.

The Real Deal

Wait. Aren't you the one with the freakishly low blood pressure?
— sTMS clinical trial facilitator

It's another emotional upturn as I get ready to head in for my first day of "off-label" treatment. It's the first day I can nest under the Eggbeater, or "Egg" as I'm told the NeoSync execs are said to call it, and know that its *rackety-rack-rack* is actually spinning magnetic waves across my cortex. In my six-week-study-concluding assessment yesterday, I'm asked all the usual questions. About self-harm, suicidal tendencies, counting, obsessing, energy, sadness, inferiority, appetite, sleep, reality and unreality. My actual upturn isn't reflected in my answers. But my tempered responses can't spare me the tests.

The battery is a repeat of those I endured at the

trial's start. There's space bar-tapping to gauge how well I recognize the letter B; a test to see if I can quickly differentiate between the word "yellow" when it's written in red, blue, green, and yellow; how many words like barn, window, church, and bird I can recall in order; and then a recall of geometric shapes like bisected squares, perpendicular lines, triangles bruised by tiny circles.

I'm asked if I think I have received the placebo these six weeks. If my symptoms have improved? Did something the facilitator say give it away? Something the principal investigator said? Something about the device itself? Though I was certain I got the placebo at the trial's start (who would design a sleek hi-tech machine like the Eggbeater and then make it sound like Chitty Chitty Bang Bang?), I was more positive now. Just getting off my meds seemed to lay the groundwork for recovery. Then I saw my emotive and energetic states changing in ways I could only explain by crediting the device.

"Wait. Aren't you the one with the freakishly low blood pressure?" the facilitator asks squinting at me playfully. It's low, but the freakish part is my pulse. She counts 48. "Normal is 60 to 80," she says. "Has it always been this low?"

"I guess it means I'm going to live to 120," I laugh.

"Yeah, you're saving them up."

Back upstairs I sign documents waiving my HIPAA protections. I'm warned as the device is wheeled into place that it is programmed to sound differently than the six-week machines. I'm told the sound doesn't mean anything. For sure, this one is more NASA and less Miss Chitty. It just sounds like it's working. As with the previous machine, there are three noises. The most unique resembles a cicada fluttering furiously in a paper bag, cellophane wings crackling with every urgent beat. Beneath that a kind of a motor driving steady and firm. There's a third I can't place easily. Ball bearings gliding, maybe, clicking over each other with muted taps.

I feel the familiar web-like spreading of nerves along my cheeks and smile.

Bottled Lightning

What wisdom can you find that is greater than kindness?

— Jean Jacques Rousseau

Inside those delicate tendrils of spider-web electricity I'm able to soften my mind and heart. Let go of the hardening I use daily in an attempt to guard myself from a world that feels so charged with violence and predation. During these breezy days of authentic treatment I focus on encouraging my kindest thoughts and accepting that my life may be a quieter one from here out. I understand and accept that my recovery may require me to limit my stress in ways that prohibit my ever having my talents, such as they are, acknowledged by any audience. It could be, as they call it, a simple life.

Maybe I'll spend my days mastering the Johnny

Cash songbook. Maybe I'll prepare, plant, and tend a garden for the first time. With no public presence to maintain, perhaps I'll reestablish my mohawk, topped off with green bandana and ball cap. I think about volunteering at the state hospital or a hospice and returning to the homeless shelter. And I can always write. Under-employment will allow for lots of that.

By the end of the third week of off-label treatment, I've grown so stir-crazy that I drop out without that last week of magnetism. I return home a bottle of lightning.

In the first two weeks I ...

- Set up a home office
- Fix a collapsed wall shelf and construct a floor shelf in my daughter's room
- Catch up on my finances
- Tune up the car
- Drag two bathtubs around the back yard to create a lettuce patch and a pond
- Sprout a tray of leafy-green seeds and transplant a dozen aloe plants and elephant ears
- Do my laundry (twice) and get my hair cut (just once)
- Install a new operating system on my home computer and fix 38 things online
- Dunk my cell phone in an irrigation ditch after following my bliss down a dreamy country road to balance my way along an old acequia

- Order a new cell phone
- Submit an Open Records request for all documents related to my part in the sTMS trial (denied) and medical files from my psychiatrist and recent therapists (released)
- Sweep and mop my house and cover the lower windows in the front of the house with brilliant obscuring colorful cellophane of various colors
- And, yeah, I scrub the toilet. More than once.

I have been a cleaning and constructing fool. I should be taking long naps and resting, but I'm unable to stop moving. I bike to the library to write most days, because at home my focus is diverted into a thousand and one different projects. Sleeping remains a problem, but it's a small price to pay. I find that I'm engaged with my surroundings in such deep ways that I'm not dwelling on my internal life much. That's new. I'm smiling, open, and singing as I move around the garden observing deeply every tree, every insect, closing my eyes to really feel each breeze.

Before I launched out on this trial business, I had a hard time doing anything, even making a bowl of cereal. Now? I'm surprised I haven't started working out recipes to make and market my own brand of morning crunch. It's like that. I frequently have to pause to sit myself down and make sure this surge of life force is creative enthusiasm and not mania. A few nights ago the spirits sat me down as well.

I dreamed:

At the fortune teller's house. I tell her how much
my daughter enjoyed visiting recently (?). She's
touched. She wants to tell our fortune in particular
way (there's someone by my side I never see who), she
says, but I object. 'No. Here,' I say, setting up a plain
chest with three items on it. Basically, it's a challenge
to her to improvise, to prevent any trickery of
prepared materials. My first question is about getting
back to work and she says, "No. You are going to get
close to nature first."

After I leave I see a taloned bird of prey high in the
sky, small and unbelievably agile. Watching its
acrobatics I jokingly hold out my arm for it to land
and someone warns me that it will tear my arm off. I
reassure them I'll pull my arm away should it go into a
dive. I pull on the elbow-length glove and someone
gets me a couple mice to hold. The hawk dives
sharply, directly, and I feel it grip my arm firmly but
without injury. It feeds.

Against the Ego

*He seems in this semiheadless state to have found a renewed vigor
and sense of purpose.*

Gordon Grice, *The Red Hourglass: Lives of the Predators*

Part of me desperately wants to go back to full-time
journalism work, to show the world I'm not that sick.
That I'm better, actually. As good as ever. That part of
me has that something to prove. Yet I know to
surrender to it, to measure myself by the opinions of
others, is a short trip back to sickness.

In this season of newness and excitement, I'm still
flooded with worry and sadness – even slip into
periodic depression (or is this what they call sadness?).
One of the key strategies I find myself utilizing to stay
healthy is a constant attention on my heart. Whenever
I'm gripped by grief or selfishness or fear, I can feel a

constriction in my chest. I've also learned to watch for that and how to soften again. To open and expand. To love in spite of whatever is going on around me, whatever the passing feeling. Each time I start to feel sick in my mind or emotions, I check in with my heart. Virtually every time the answer is opening, loving, and accepting.

Thanks to my rekindled energy and my heart mediation I can feel a new me emerging. I catch myself thinking that this is the person I always knew I could be. The one I've been waiting for. This is why I'd held on for all these years. If I have learned nothing else through this adventure, if there is no other thing I can put into practice in my remaining days, it is to be patient with myself. To forgive and to be patient.

Left to Wonder

If we aspire to contribute something to our society — to achieve a new vision of things — we need to begin with ourselves.

— Matthieu Ricard, *Destructive Emotions: How Can We Overcome Them?*

My energetic rush, a generative vitality I hadn't felt in many years, continued for about two months. While I came out of the trial in far better shape than I went in, an inevitable retrenchment followed. An incremental return of brooding and ambivalence. "The whole concept of TMS is still theoretical. However, data would clearly suggest that the technology works," John Carnuccio, CEO of NeoSync, told me in a brief email exchange. "Duration is an uncertain, an unknown."

Rhodes suffered a relapse, too, but pulled out with

10 TMS treatments and now receives TMS twice a month for maintenance, she said. She's not an anomaly. "Based on my experience, there's probably a third of people who will relapse and need additional treatments," one Texas-based psychiatrist told me. "If we catch them early, we can sometimes get them back with three to 15 treatments." I can only assume the same must hold for sTMS.

I signed on for a couple weeks of rTMS at an area clinic as my previous disorder began to lock back into place, but nothing changed. Though my parents offer to pay for more treatments, I'm not willing to bank their generosity on such a costly uncertainty.

It was the student of Chinese medicine who, after checking the color of my tongue and skin, suggested I cut out wheat for a month and increase my water intake. A noticeable improvement followed. The addition of a low dose of bipolar medication further stretched what had become weekly cycles. Have I been misdiagnosed my whole life? Is this so-called "unipolar" depression nagging on my heels? And the absolute strangeness of my depressed mind to my healthy one, the healthy mind's disbelief that depression could ever return: was this some mild form of schizophrenia? These much-debated divisions have lost interest to me. All live on a spectrum. All are to be observed, noted, and let go of. To obsess is only to magnify their hold.

I am left to wonder when, or if, the Eggbeater will be cleared for use: a device I know to work. Carnuccio wrote to confirm his company is indeed seeking clearance to begin marketing the Eggbeater (though certainly by another name). He added that since depression tends to be a "lifelong" condition he hoped the machine will be one people can check out from their doctor's offices for self-administered daily home treatments. "It's a pretty simple device," he said. "It can be done in most hands, but not everyone's hands. But that's our objective." Unfortunately, officials at the FDA won't tell me when or if they will consider the company's request.

The Eggbeater and the growing number of devices like it do quite a lot, I've found. If Dr. Persinger's high-frequency fields truly do create "ghosts" in the mind, the lower-frequencies provided by TMS appear equally capable of dispelling them.

At least much of the time. For a time.

Beginning, Enduring

The blade that whirls at the gates of Eden is not our enemy. It
protects Eden and it protects us.

– Evan Eisenberg, *The Ecology of Eden*

The sky has opened up over the city. Daily
rainstorms are manifesting new rivers, revealing
unknown channels, swamping cars, sweeping streets,
and rushing in sheets across fields and parking lots,
cement ditches, and grass-pocked slopes. To the north,
they are stealing bodies, taking houses. The deluge
herds waves of plastic, that urban crust, into the ever-
accepting downstream. Gaping mouths in the rock
sputter and choke, swallowing what they are able,
funneling the sudden overpowering riches into
subterranean seas inhabited by albino spiders and
creamy eyeless salamanders before passing them

further still into lightless calm and noiselessness.

This tantrum of the skies, this light and thunder, is a comfort. Accustomed as we are in South Texas to a steady sun, reliable heat, and sky of perpetual blue and billowing white, this reasserted dominance chasing us indoors, away from bridges and off the land, is shaking awake previously dormant fears of flood and funnel cloud, of being swallowed alive. It's an important reminder for small creatures like us who grip the earth with frail impermanent pincers. It tells me my own innate destructiveness is elemental, celestial.

To track and even interrupt these storms takes focus. When the energetic body flags, conscious creation. In the year since my magnetic gains slipped away, I've consulted the acupuncturist, deepened my meditation, and taught myself some basic qigong movements, a dance with openhandedness at its heart. You don't grasp, the greatest teachings tell us. You hold and cherish and pass along.

With bare feet pressing in heavily trafficked floorboards, I lift my bare arms above me as the winds lean against the front of our house. I feel the room breathe with the sky. I draw in this universal energy and push it, palms down, into the earth as if directing the ungraspable forces of the sky. There is nothing that isn't swept up, that isn't battered and dragged down. Nothing that doesn't return. In this moving meditation, I gather the energy around me and guide it through as a cleansing. I am working to fill this place with power—to pass it through, with the intention of easing the suffering of another in some undetermined way. I'm pained by how little I know about the forces around me. My consistent inability to speak to shared sufferings and dispel them. But in the gathering darkness and streaks of blinding light, I am overwhelmed by a strange serenity.

I know now what I must do.

Further Reading

Anatomy Of An Epidemic: Magic Bullets, Psychiatric Drugs, And The Astonishing Rise of Mental Illness in America
Robert Whitaker
Broadway Paperbacks, 2010

Buddha's Nature: A Practical Guide to Enlightenment Through Evolution
Wes Nisker
Bantam Books, 1998

Destructive Emotions: How We Overcome Them (A Scientific Dialogue With The Dalai Lama)
Daniel Goleman
Bantam Books, 2003

Malignant Sadness: The Anatomy Of Depression
Lewis Wolpert
Free Press, 1999

The Balance Within: The Science Connecting Health And Emotions
Esther M. Sternberg
W. H. Freeman And Company, 2000

The Body Electric: Electromagnetism And The Foundation Of Life
Robert O. Becker & Gary Selden
William Morrow and Company, 1985

The Brain That Changes Itself: Stories of Personal Triumph from the Frontiers of Brain Science
Norman Doidge
Penguin Books, 2007

The Energy Healing Experiments: Science Reveals Our Natural Power To Heal
Gary Schwartz
Atria Books, 2007

The Wisdom of Depression: A Guide To Understanding And Curing Depression Using Natural Medicine
Jonathan Zuess
Harmony Books, 1998

Three Thousand Pulses Later: A Memoir of Surviving Depression Without Medication
Martha Rhodes
Pushpin Press, 2013

Unhinged: The Trouble With Psychiatry — A Doctor's Revelations About A Profession In Crisis
Daniel J. Carlat
Free Press, 2010

Vibrational Medicine for the 21st Century: A Complete Guide To Energy Healing And Spiritual Transformation
Richard Gerber
William Morrow, 2000

Where To Find Help

If you have a mental health emergency, dial 911 (U.S. and Canada) or 999 or 112 (United Kingdom).

Canadian Mental Health Association
Direct service to more than 100,000 Canadians each year.
1110-151 Slater Street
Ottawa, ON K1P 5H3
(416) 977-5580
cmha.ca

The Icarus Project
Support network by and for people who experience the world in ways that are often diagnosed as mental illness.
theicarusproject.net

Mental Health America
Leading community-based non-profit dedicated to helping all Americans achieve wellness by living mentally healthier lives.
2000 N. Beauregard Street
6th Floor Alexandria, VA 22311
(800) 969-6642
mentalhealthamerica.net

Mental Health Foundation
UK's leading mental health charity.
Colechurch House
1 London Bridge Walk
London SE1 2SX
+44 (0)20 7803 1100
mentalhealth.org.uk

Mad In America
A resource and community for those interested in rethinking psychiatric care in the United States and abroad.
madinamerica.com

The National Alliance on Mental Illness
Grassroots mental health organization dedicated to building better lives for those affected by mental illness.
3803 N. Fairfax Drive, Ste 100
Arlington, VA 22203
(800) 950-6264 (Help Line)
nami.org

www.ingramcontent.com/pod-product-compliance
Lightning Source LLC
Chambersburg PA
CBHW070900180526
45168CB00005B/1883